The Enemy

by

Colin Biggs

©

Gloucester Edition published by:

Pipers' Ash

www.supamasu.com

CHIPPENHAM   WILTSHIRE   ENGLAND

SN15 4BW

Dedicated to Roseanna Biggs
My loving grandmother, who always had a job for me
and never let me get away with anything
(this made me the man I am today).

Acknowledgments
Zoe Jackson, for typing my notes in the early days.
My wife Jacqueline, who puts up with me.
And everybody who gave me the encouragement to
move forward and put pen to paper.

'Gloucester Edition'
ISBN 978-1-904494-78-2

Contents

Page

PREFACE

I HAVE MS and am looking forward to the rest of my life! This book is not just about me, although it is my story, my life and thoughts, ideas I have tried, along with the help and advice from others, but it is for every MS sufferer, especially the newly diagnosed, their families and carers.

I hope you will find this mixed up bag of thoughts useful, as nothing like this was available to me when I was first diagnosed, they just said its MS and that's it. But that's not it, it is far from it as you can get. I didn't let others try and make decisions for me, as its my life and I am in the driving seat, so look out I am coming down the street, don't step out in front of me. This is what has encouraged me to put this story in writing, so others may benefit from and may be empathise with the state of MS to be endured.

I had to spend hours and hours drudging through endless boring books and articles, each one pointing the way I should go to elevate the symptoms. I have since found that there is not sufficient time left in my life to try all the so called remedies with any degree of success, so it's my call and my call only, except none of the effort would be possible without the support and encouragement from my wife Jacqueline (she's a brick). Its me who directly lives with the condition (others indirectly) and only me who knows how I feel, so question any advice given but don't be dependent upon it.

I have titled this book, The Enemy Within 'because that's what its like. If you try to quickly to speed up any form of recovery, the MS will find out what your doing and as an enemy to your body, turn on you as quick as a rat up a drain pipe. Then the likely outcome is a deterioration in your condition, its one step forward and two steps back if you try to rush any progress.

I resolved to look the disease right in the face, peer deep into the abyss. I knew that I couldn't fight and win the war against MS but I could win some of the battles and encourage it to become an ally but an ally to be wary of. There is no cure. No one has ever beaten MS in a straight fight, no matter who claims what. The one weapon needed on your journey through the forthcoming swamp of endless crap is PMA, (positive mental attitude). Without it you haven't a snowballs chance in hell of being able to put up any sort of a fight and you will certainly fall at the first hurdle.

For me, the key was, though I couldn't beat MS, but I wouldn't be beaten either.

That seemed to me to be how to treat MS. It's here to stay but it's not the end by any means. It's not even the beginning of the end. My life can go on. Maybe things have to be a little different, but they will go on nonetheless.

One thing you must not do is think of what you can't do, that's a negative view of your life and anything negative puts you on the defensive. There is numerous things you will be able to do, just take a leaf out of Danny Wallace's book. He's the gentleman who used to play for Manchester United who is now an MS sufferer and walked the London marathon. This major feat took him seven days to complete, falling occasionally but he did it and what a good positive view that is of what you can do.

At the end of the day it all comes down to your choice, as you are in the front line with MS. We all treat our bodies with contempt, our car has an MOT test every year to make sure it is safe and our house requires regular repair and decoration to maintain its value. But we just neglect ourselves no matter what, until we break down, then the hard work starts trying to build ourselves up.

Dr Choy from the MS Healing Trust described it as 20% MS and 80% muscle wastage due to a lack of use. But remember as yet there is no cure for MS and no two people are alike and no two conditions are the same, what works for one does not work for another. All I say is try and give it your best shot, but most of all, believe in yourself. The first thing you must do is to be your doctors friend (because you are going to need all the support there is) and talk to him or her, to make sure that they know just what you are about to do, as this may interfere with any medication you are currently taking.

Do not forget, we will die with MS but not because of it. Treat the covers of this book as goal posts and use it as a tool to try and find your goal. As starting points on the road to finding what will work for you, may I suggest the following:-* Reduce your stress level immediately.

* Rest when your body tells you (don't be a hero)
* Try to keep on a healthy low fat diet.
* Regular gentle exercise, both physical and mental.
* You will certainly need a good nights sleep (rest lets your body build up energy)
* For me, avoiding increases of ambulant temperature (I will explain further on)
* Become a member of the MS Society, the largest organisation for help.
* For the most up to date information, use the Internet (I am lost without it), then you are off to try and find your goal in the maze of so-called specialist advice.

Some questions you all want answers to:

* Will I die from MS? Not likely, all depends on how the MS acted and what nerves are damaged.
* Will I go blind? Not likely, all depends on how the MS acted and what nerves are damaged.
* Will I be able to drive? Yes, automatic and hand controls are available, all depends on how the MS acted and what nerves are damaged to the adaptations you may require.
* Will I need a wheelchair? All depends on how the MS acted and what nerves are damaged.
* Can I have a family? Most likely MS has never been a barrier to having and raising a family, you adapt.
* Will I loose my job? No, all employers must make allowances for employees with a disability, it's the law.

So you can see that MS is not an exact science, there is so many variables and answers to the questions you may wish to ask. So don't think the worse, there's no need, all you will succeed in doing is worry needlessly to something know one really knows the answer to with any conviction.

The only chapter I failed to write myself, although I tried but felt myself far from qualified to offer an educated answer, was on religious faith. This is a very personal part of ones life, beliefs and hopes, though pray may offer support and comfort in so many ways to the individual concerned. So I called upon Silvia Quirk, a woman I met whilst swimming, who recognised me from a local press article and knew I was writing about MS. Her testimony to the power of faith is chapter eleven.

ABOUT THE AUTHOR

My name is Colin Biggs! Who am I? I have MS and I am looking forward to the rest of my life as an adventure. My story starts on the 7th of May 1951. That's when I popped out at the maternity hospital, alive and kicking, the first son of Alf and Reenie Biggs. I eventually became the middle child in a family of three, having on older sister Pauline and a younger brother George. George is two years younger, still a bachelor (he has his head screwed on right) and helps with jobs around the house and garden, as I would be totally lost without his help and encouragement. I had a reasonably happy childhood, getting into all kinds of mischief as boys do and getting a regular belting from my dad when he found out. Like playing with a magnifying glass on a bright sunny day, I set fire to next doors door curtain, which they used to guard the paintwork against the sun (I had a bloody good belting for that one). Life was tough in the fifties, no money but we made do, not like nowadays, where your more likely to be mugged or your property vandalised. We would play rolling an old car tyre down the street, use an empty bean tin playing "tin can nurky" or draw wickets on a wall to play cricket. It was all harmless fun and kept you from under your mothers feet. I used to play on the nearby old disused allotments with a handful of my mates. We would build a gang hut out of old tin sheets and anything else we could find, then put car seats in it and it was our gang HQ. Money, who needed money! There wasn't any to be had, so we all just entertained ourselves for free, getting shit up in the process.

I was six years old and it was the end of the long school holiday so we were all ready to go back to school. We all had our new clothes and shoes (jumble sale stuff really but it was new to us, NO DESIGNER GEAR HERE) then to top it all, I fell ill and couldn't go back to school. I had contracted jaundice and was as yellow as a banana, the doctor said six weeks off school my boy, which meant twelve weeks in all. After the first week I started to feel ok , wrong thing to be, my Gran had me doing every little job she could, digging the garden, cutting the grass, picking apples off the tree and worsted of all, painting the bedroom I was to later move in to. As jaundice is infectious, no friends were allowed to see me, this was a buggar as I was becoming fed up, time off school is good but not on your own. Kids in the street called me china man as the yellow was quite bright and said I would soon have slant eyes, stupid sods!

At the age of seven, I was moved into Gran's due to the fact my parents only managed to buy a two-bedroom house which as it turned out was there one and only step on the property ladder. So I spent my formative years living with my maternal grandmother Rosie, who spoiled me as much as I helped her, it was good living there, I had my own room, and my own space in the world (she is the person to who I owe for providing me with the knowledge to become a man). I didn't mind helping her really, I rather enjoyed it, as I treated the garden as my own and began to grow flowers and veg. The other thing about living with gran was the egg round on a Saturday morning. My father kept chickens, well rather a lot actually, about two hundred. He used to take the eggs to work and sell them, the ones left over would go to Grans house and she would take orders which were delivered by me on a Saturday.

I was groomed in the art of selling, I had to take the eggs, knock on the door, hold my hand out and say "my grandma Rosie has sent the eggs and they are five shillings a dozen" and not to return empty handed. That was just part of the weekend, the best bit was Saturday night. My Gran and I would watch the telly eating fresh home made bread and she would give me half a bottle of Mackison stout, brought on a Saturday morning by her brother, my uncle Charlie. I felt very grown up and important.

At the age of twelve I joined the Scouts, which was one of the best moves I have ever made in my life. My scout leader Jack was a very straight talking down to earth sort of guy. He talked to you on the same level, which seemed to give you confidence in your abilities. We used to go on camp, which meant participating and learning all kinds of woodcraft, which for me was the tools and knowledge I required for later life out on the fells. I became a patrol leader, which gave me the responsibility for six lads and I remember once winning a cooking competition, (that was more luck that skill). I loved the freedom that scouting gave me and I eventually became a Queen Scout, representing the town at various gatherings.

Weekends, school holidays etc, I was off camping in the Lake District with my school friend Jim. We would get all over the place looking for a nights shelter and sometimes food. I have seen us eating fodder thrown out by the farmer for his sheep, "buggar the sheep we were hungry". I was only fourteen at the time, my parents trusted me not to get into any more trouble, which I didn't and with their encouragement it felt good to be away from home, I was never one for sitting in front of the telly anyhow. Parents are more protective of their children nowadays, which is a shame really as my time out and about looking after myself was a great character builder and I believe it prepared me for later life. At the age of fifteen I moved back home, as my sister had married, moved into her own house. This was a bit of a shock to the system and meant no more spoiling for Col, but it was better really as I used to be out late in the evening, which was not fair on my Gran.

I somehow (don't ask me how) eventually grew into a practical steady hardworking adult. I had a secondary school education, leaving at the age of 16 with a handful of CSE's, which I have never required since, so that was a waste of my time and theirs, but my dad wanted me to stay on at school, so there you go. All my friends left school when they were 15 and started work in jobs like delivering the Co-op milk or office boys in the shipyard or town hall. My Dad thought if I stayed on at school I might better myself, but I knew what I wanted and it didn't involve school.

I used to spend my spare time stripping down and rebuilding old car engines in our back yard. They were given to me by one of our scout instructors, they were scrap really but I had to start somewhere. I was fascinated by the technology and science of the internal combustion engine, so the motor trade seemed destined to be my first career.

The day I started work, I vowed that I would never be skint again and I haven't been, there is always a way to make honest cash.

Mostly, my working life consisted of manual work as my first job was working for British Steel in the local wire works, this was a hard shitty job but enjoyable at the same time. I was making money and it felt good to have coin in my pocket. I worked a two-shift system, 6am to 2pm and 2pm to 10pm and the wage was £7 a week. The late shift played hell with my social life, as I was going out with Glenis my first steady girlfriend at that time. That relationship only lasted the summer of 1967 (well you don't only shop at one store do you), she was a lovely girl and I was a complete bastard to her. You know how it is, trying to get everything you can but not really knowing what you are going to do with it when you get it (I often wondered what happened to her, until I found her on the Internet I am now in contact, via e-mail and she has forgiven me for being a right bastard).

I left the Wire works after twelve weeks and used some of the money to go on holiday. I went to the world scout jamboree in America for three weeks, my friend David and I were the only two to go from Barrow and we had a ball. We stayed in Idaho for the jamboree and then to Denver Colorado, having hospitality with a fireman called Harold and his family. (I wonder if that was the reason I finally ended up in that profession) This is another person who I am now in contact with via the Internet; you can't hide in this world anymore.

On my return, I started my first career and served my apprenticeship as a diesel fitter at a local haulage contractor, which was like out of the frying pan and right into the fire. At the time, working on heavy goods vehicles was slave labour, no proper washing facilities and more shit than the job before, all for £5 a week. My mother used to play hell at the state of my working clothes as they stunk of oil and had to be washed separately. Money, I had money. Let me see, a motor bike, that's it my own transport and independence. So I went and bought a Triumph Tiger Cub for £65.00 (I was a bit skint till it was paid off), my first wheels but definitely not my last. Then I needed a car, somewhere warm and out of the cold and rain. A bloke down the street was selling his old 1953 Morris Oxford, a bit of a shed but it had an MOT, so with a bit of pleading poverty and promising I would look after his old girl we came to a price, £5,00 but it cost me £20.00 to insure it. I was the proud owner of a car, a bit oily and it through out a bit of smoke but it was mine.

I finished serving my time and with a handful of qualifications, I moved to two other garages but it was the same shit but different places. The skills I gained made me a good living on the side as I had a flair for making money, it felt good to have cash in my pocket. I was always fixing cars and at one time I had so much work coming in, that I opened a small garage and paid Bob an old mate of mine cash in hand just to cope with the extra work. (sadly he's dead now, living a life of fags and drink) The extra money I made came in very handy, so I started to buy and sell cars, which I bought at the auctions, this made me more cash. I suppose I became a dodgy car salesman, someone you could trust (I don't think so, but I think my heart was in the right place).

I had a steady girlfriend at the time and being a flash bastard with cars, motorbikes and money, I had a rush of blood to the brain and thought marriage would be a good thing to do next (big mistake, that soon started to suck the cash out of my pocket).

I married her in December 1972, a lovely girl but later found out (too bloody late really)not a loving wife, she carried more emotional baggage from her family life than even she could deal with at times. Our first house as a little two bedroom terrace which cost £4.000.00 and it took me and my dad nine months to get it into liveable order. I was mister DIY, fitting gas fires, upstairs toilet and rewiring, couldn't do it now, too many regulations and red tape. In October 1975 our first daughter Nichola was born (who is now a schoolteacher) and then in November 1977 our second daughter Lindsey, where I attended the birth and a moving experience it was (she is now a midwife) and I was a proud farther of two lovely girls. The girls were going to need their own space, as they shared a bedroom, so we moved to a bigger house with a basement games room and garage. This move was very beneficial, I could work on cars at home in my spare time and was making money hand over fist.

It was at this time I realised that the spark had gone out of my job and it was not enough to satisfy me anymore. I was fed up of being shit up all the time and at twenty six years old I wanted more family security and a good pension in later life, as the motor trade being a young mans job with few prospects had little to offer anymore.

It was the winter of 1977 and the firemen were on strike fighting for better pay and conditions. A few of my friends were firemen and the sense of working for the community and perhaps saving the odd life or two appealed to me   This give me the shove I wanted, where upon I joined the Cumbria Fire Service in May 1978, working in Barrow, which was a major career change but still a manual occupation. (less shit)

I enjoyed a reasonably happy married life and with our daughters we all had fantastic holidays and a good standard of living. Life was good, I had the career I wanted and also started to lecture on motor vehicle maintenance part time at the local college. This again brought in extra cash, which was spent on family holidays. In 1988 I was promoted to Leading Fireman, on a day manned station on Walney Island, which meant moving again. This move proved harder as we had difficulty selling our house so I had to sleep alone on the station for six months before we completed, (it was like being single again). In September 1990 I was up the ranks again as Sub Officer but the downside was I had to travel to Carlisle. I must have been doing something right because two months later I was on my way up again to Station Officer. I worked in Carlisle for eleven months before transferring back to Barrow, where

I stayed until I retired. We were a normal functional family unit (or so I thought).

Some of the funny story's I have come across in the Fire Service as they happened to me are unbelievable. To put it in a nutshell, common sense is a must if you want to be a good fireman and if you have none, "well" you are going to have the piss taken out of you constantly. There was one incident that comes to mind, where the upstairs of a terrace house was well alight. I asked Mick a fireman to KNOCK the power off. He thought about it and went and immediately picked up a sledge hammer to start to knock the electric meter off the wall, "thick bastard" he could have injured himself, not to mention me. (knock the power off indeed, he took the words literally, thick sod no common sense). Another time we were having a drill on a ship at the local dock's, I ordered Stuart to throw the line (rope) down so a fire hose could be hauled up to the deck of the ship. To my amazement that's just what he did, "thick shit", he threw the whole thing down without tying it off first. This sort of thing happened all the time and it always will, a fireman is just a council worker when all said and done. But it is the best job in the world, full of laugh's and funny incidents.

My hobbies ranged from scouting, where I became a Queen Scout and gained a taste of the adventurous life, living outdoors with only me and the earth to contend with. Then I tried motor X riding (where I was off the bike more times than on it), landing up in the local hospital with concussion and begging them not to cut my leathers off because they were new and expensive. This was a very expensive pastime due to the cost of engine rebuilds and other maintenance. I also had a young family to support at the time. So motor X only lasted three years, the family came first.

Potholing was the next adventure (which was sometimes done at night after a skin full of ale) which wet my appetite for risk and adventure, as you were in a dangerous situation some of the time (never told the misses about them, what you don't know won't hurt you). On one occasion I had to use my car and tow an old school friend Rob out of a mineshaft, called Pylon Pot. Silly buggar was too fat and unfit, but we all laughed about it in the pub later, while he licked his wounds.

I was once working on a car, getting it ready for its MOT (it was a knacker but it scraped through). When I produced the MOT certificate to the owner, the cheeky bastard said he was grateful for the work I'd done but sorry as he had no money to pay me at the present time. At this, I blew my top and took the two complete sets of scuba gear which was in the boot of the car. I told him he could have the gear back when he paid me, he never did pay me, so I became the proud owner of scuba gear, and this was the start of another adventure hobby. I gave a set of scuba gear to my friend Ray, so we set upon an adventure under the water, this hobby you can't do alone. The scuba diving was a bit risky, as it was you and buggar all else between life and death at 100 ft below the surface, but I survived that one as well. We found allsorts under the water, old bottles and plates, numerous fishing spinners and the best find of all, was two outboard motors, which I repaired and sold (I split the cash with Ray).

But after all that excitement, my one true love was walking, climbing and hiking throughout the British Isles with my Fire Service colleagues and my Lakeland Terrier dog Bess. The thing with that was, as long as you carried a map and compass and knew how to use them (scouting again) you won't be calling out the mountain rescue when you get lost, like the city slickers do. We trod over all the fells and mountains in the lakes, travelled to Scotland where we used crampons and ice axe, for our winter safety and we all supported each other when we were away, especially in the pub afterwards.

It was on one of these walks that I noticed that I began to drag my right foot and lost control of the movement to put it down onto the ground. This seemed to be short lived because it only seemed to happen when I was extremely tired and after exerting myself (which meant my body was hot). When it became more frequent I consulted a locum GP and was told to take paracetamol and see how it went! (This was probably the only advice I could have expected, as the condition was in its infancy).

As a consequence to me being promoted to Station Officer, I had to spend quite a considerable amount of time studying at the Fire Service College in Moreton-in-Marsh, Gloucestershire, where I met three very good friends. Jim, who came from Dunfermline in Scotland (sadly he passed away after a heart condition), Mike, who lives in Belfast, Northern Ireland and Roy from Newcastle. We all used to meet every year, taking it in turns to be the host, for a weekend on the beer, having a bet on the horses, where we won quite a bit and having a general good chat and piss take. Mike, Roy and I still meet up at my house, as I find it very difficult to travel on my own any more, but we are still connected. The Fire Service College was a blessing in disguise, as I could rest frequently, especially on my last visit to the college which was a twelve week course learning Fire Safety. That course involved attending lectures and I was able to hide my progressive tired condition with the MS was still trying to find its own level. Students began to notice that I was walking around in my short sleeved uniform shirt and this was in the middle of winter. I used to say that my thermostat wasn't working, but the truth was that the cold made me feel better and my walking improved. This is still true today as I am in tee shirts and shorts in the house, use the air conditioning in the car in Winter and just feel less fatigued when I am cooler. When I returned from college, I was trying every trick in the book to enable me to continue undetected. As time pasted, my balance became affected, I began to trip and stumble frequently and I was dragging my right leg more and more. I would walk 200 metres from my home to the local shop, but on my way back I was staggering as if drunk, due to fatigue and the erratic gait in my walking. On one Sunday morning, my neighbour Gordon thought I was pissed and said jokingly, it's a bit early in the day to be in that state Colin. This led me to again seek professional advice, as being thought of as a pisshead was even too much for me to cope with at the time. However, this time after two MRI scans, the diagnosis was positive, it's MS my boy. This was a relief of some kind, I always believed the worst, (so did some of my work colleagues) as I thought I had Motor Neurone Disease, which we all know is more disabling and terminal. At work, I used to say that I had twisted my ankle or that my leg was sore due to a pulled muscle, but finally after a further twelve months working I knew it was time to say enough is enough and forced myself to go on sick leave. The final nail in the coffin was when I was inspecting a local hotel for its fire certificate, I tripped and landed flat on my face in the street. That in itself didn't seem so bad, but it was pissing it down with rain at the time, I broke my fall with my hands, cutting them badly and all my files were spread across the street. I knew it was the end. The decision was made for me, the bastard MS had halted my career!

My wife and I lived with the biggest secret of our lives, as we knew it would affect the whole family unit and also my career. We needed to comprehend the situation we found ourselves in before sharing it with other people. Both Nichola and Lindsey were at Liverpool University and I vowed nothing was going to rock their boat, life was just beginning for them. However in 1996 after eighteen months on sick leave, I eventually retired from the Fire Service and the secret was out.

After retiring I sat at home in a kind of shock and grief for what I had lost. I read constantly about MS, how the disease could progress and wondered what was to become of me! My worries ranged from financial matters, future security and even to my own independence but most of all, what was going to happen to the family?

I decided that moping around was not for me, as it is all to simple to just give up and become a couch potato, so after a swift kick up the arse from those close to me at the time, I looked for a voluntary position I could do sitting down.

I enrolled in a local disability organization and successfully completed a series of computer courses gaining RSA qualifications. This encouraged me to attend a foundation credit course with Lancaster University, which gave me the required twenty credits to progress to a degree course (which is on hold at the moment). I then became Chairman of the same disability organization and trained as a Welfare Benefits Adviser. I soon became aware that I was not alone and there were other people far more disabled that myself who lived life to the full.

I was offered a place on a foundation credit course from Lancaster University, which in its self seemed a positive move forward. The course was split into modules to make it a bit easer for the disabled students and it was. An enterprise module was the last project and it was decided by the four students involved (one being myself) to open a charity shop for six weeks. That was way back in 1998 and today that shop is still open and has another outlet in a different part of the town. The shops fund local disability organisations including a local benefits advice centre and Shopmobility outlet, offering scooters and wheelchair hire. Also, I am proud to say that the shops have been granted registered charity status and we now offer holidays to disabled people in our own fully adapted holiday home. I am now secretary of the new charity, which is The Thrift Charitable Trust, help run the benefits advice service and looking forward to future enterprises the charity is working on.

In March 2001 my life was rocked when my 29 year marriage ended, leaving for someone else who wasn't disabled, (when future prospects are bleak, love goes out the fucking window and its then that you need the love and support of a partner, which I never had)

My children had grown up, obtained good careers and formed their own lives. Once again I wondered what was to become of me, as all attempts at reconciliation with my wife had failed. I was devastated and could not believe that my life had become so fragile to the point that my condition had worsened due to the stress of the matrimonial collapse. Its times like this that makes you wonder who your true friends are. A true friend of mine is Graham, a Fire Service chum, has taken me on holiday a few times to try and stop the rot setting in. We travelled to France and Spain, most of the time we were both pissed but great holidays and great fun. Those who I thought would stick by me, slowly drifted away as they were accepting of what my ex wife had done and they could now socialise together with her new partner. By this time I was quite dependant upon the wheelchair for my outside mobility, I was dying inside and became dependant on other people to help me. It was at this time that Social Services stepped in and offered me personal care to get up in the morning and in the words of Ricky Tomlinson, it was life my arse!

However, by chance, my life again took another turn and I met up with Jacqueline, a young woman I had known for many years. She was living with her two daughters after having been divorced and we just seem to click together. MS was something she knew nothing about and it was me she began to love, the MS was part of the package. I am now happily living in that new partnership with a new family unit, having married in March 2003 and once again having two lovely daughters, Katie and Sarah. My life has a new direction, with added vitality and I am using the wheelchair less and less, as I now have increased self-motivation and feel loved and wanted as never before. I now have a reason to live life to the full.

What If? What If? What If? And Why Me? Why Me? Why Me?

These are the questions that goes through everybody's mind, whether they acquire disabled or not and this can bring on depression, drag you down and loose the friends who you will need. The fact of the matter is it is you and the sooner you come to terms with it, the quicker you can develop a life for yourself. Stop wallowing in self pity and grab MS by the balls. The old saying, Life's a bastard then you die is the biggest crock of shit I have ever heard, who ever made up that statement wants putting up against a wall and shooting. All right, you might think I am a cleaver bastard for me to say that and I know sometimes its hard to motivate yourself, but there is nothing like a swift kick up the arse and a few home truths to get you going, I know it happened to me.

Tell your mind what you want to do, not the other way around!

In my time I have destroyed so many toilet seats, just by flopping down on them, I have totally wrecked the shower cubicle at home, having collapsed inside it and Jacqueline ripping it apart to get me out and I can still laugh about it.

The paramedics have picked me up off the floor so many times, they are thinking of inviting me to their Christmas party. Social Services have now given me an emergency lifting cushion to try and get my arse off the floor, it's a laugh in itself, just putting it together, but it is a good help really. So you see, I am not a saint, I get pissed off regularly and shake my fist just like Basil Faulty, but that's the relief valve we all need at times no matter who you are. If you can see the funny side of things and you don't hurt yourself, well I tell you now, life is never dull in our house.

1 INTRODUCTION

Multiple Sclerosis!
What does it mean for you?
MS ,MS, what will it do?
When will I know if the MS is true?
Help, Help, my system is under attack
Please, just give me my body back

AUTOIMMUNE DISORDERS

Autoimmune disorders are immune system breakdowns. Immune defences develop what amounts to severe memory loss; which means that they no longer recognise themselves. The result is that they run amok, making auto-antibodies that attack their own tissues. These warlike autoantibodies think they are protecting their environment, but in reality they are destroying their own organs and inciting inflammatory responses. Examples of autoimmune disease include Rheumatoid Arthritis, Lupus, ME (Chronic Fatigue Syndrome/Epstein-Barr), Multiple Sclerosis, and Amyotrophic Lateral Sclerosis (ALS/Lou Gehrig's Disease).

Before we get started, here are a few basic facts. All autoimmune diseases are closely related, with the same underlying causes of over-toxicity, virus, mycoplasma or bacteria infections, and they are similar in how they affect the body. An autoimmune condition may manifest as Multiple Sclerosis in one person or ME (chronic fatigue) in someone else. Because of different genetics, or who knows what, what applies to chronic fatigue, almost always has some bearing on Multiple Sclerosis too, until they fork off and go their separate ways.

MULTIPLE SCLEROSIS: AN INTRODUCTION

* There are approximately 85,000 cases in the UK (and rising) and 2. 5 million worldwide.

* MS is a disease of the central nervous system

* About twice as many women as men have MS
* It is usually diagnosed when people are in their 20's and 30's

* MS is unpredictable; symptoms can come and go

* MS may be incurable but that doesn't mean untreatable

* Only about one in four people diagnosed with MS will ever need to use a wheelchair

* Everyone's MS is different

You're told you've got MS. What thoughts go through your mind? Probably a wheelchair? Loss of independence? Severe disability? Premature death? Worries about family, work, money? (I know, it happened to me)

The majority of people with MS will NEVER need a wheelchair and people with MS can still expect to have a good experience of life, love, marriage, children and a career.

With sound, positive information, by getting the right treatments and help from health and social care professionals, by using the support available and most important support and reassurance from your family, MS need not be the devastating diagnosis that many people imagine.

What is Multiple Sclerosis?

MS is the most common disease of the central nervous system (CNS) affecting young adults. "Sclerosis" refers to the scarring, or lesions, which occur in the CNS; and "Multiple" to the sites of damage. These may be the eye nerves, the spinal cord at mid neck level and areas around the cavities of the brain.

The CNS comprises the brain and spinal cord, which, together with the nerves connecting to the rest of the body, form the body's communication network. In MS, damage occurs to the myelin sheath, which protects the nerves in a way similar to the insulating material around an electric wire. This damage, or demyelination, alters the way messages, or nerve impulses, are conducted to and from the brain and hence disrupts functions of the body. It can be described as similar to a detour on a road; the signals in the CNS take a different and longer way to find their way to where they are needed and when they finally arrive there is no power left, thus your movement reactions are slower. The symptoms experienced will depend on the position and extent of the lesions within the CNS and most people will only experience a few symptoms.

What are the common symptoms?

*   Blurred or double vision
*   Loss of vision in one eye
*   Fatigue
*   Weakness of limbs/pins and needles
*   Poor co-ordination/balance
*   Bladder problems
*   Problems with speech/memory

What causes MS?

Basically the official line is that no one knows what causes MS – which is why there are almost as many theories as there are people with MS! Research on this suggests MS develops as a combination of factors which all have to come together in a certain way over a set period of time.

In sequence it looks something like this:

* A genetic weakness (or 'predisposition' as the doctors call it)

* A long-term nutritional deficiency or imbalance (possibly due to malabsorption)

* A long-term situation of emotional stress or strain (possibly coupled with a very specific emotional trauma)

* A severe infection, particularly of the throat (such as tonsillitis or glandular fever)

* A physical trauma or injury (this could be something dramatic such as whiplash but it could just as easily be something as simple and non-specific as falling off a chair: these sort of minor injuries often go undiagnosed and untreated because there is little or no pain and so the person injured this way doesn't think of it as an injury.)
Often it is the emotional and physical trauma together that is the straw that almost literally breaks the camel's back and brings on the first symptoms of MS.

> *Please don't assume because I look well*
> *That I feel well. Looks can be very deceiving.*
> *Many days I look great, but feel terrible and*
> *when I look like shit, please don't tell me.*

2 DIAGNOSIS

Do you know what is wrong with you?
You might be one of the chosen few
Do you wonder why it had to be you?
"I do not want to be part of the chosen few"

HOW IS MS DIAGNOSED?

One of the frustrations surrounding diagnosis is the length of time it can take. Firstly, it is a case of ruling out other possibilities, and, secondly, many neurologists prefer to wait for a second attack, relapse, or for symptoms to develop before giving a definite diagnosis. In my case, my condition slowly deteriorated without having a relapse, which is called primary progressive. It actually took two years before I was told that I had better prepare myself for the worst, as MS was the positive diagnosis. (I thought it was motor neurone disease, so I was in a way relieved that it was MS)

Clinical History

First and foremost, certain diagnosis is based on a history of symptoms - perhaps an unexplained episode of blurred vision years before, or pins and needles in the hands or feet. (In my case, I had an eye problem when I was 22 years old and at 26 years old, I had severe concussion due to a motorcycle accident. The latter I believe was the final trigger to my MS. It then lay dormant for the next twelve years and then it slowly started to progress, effecting my co-ordination and balance until mobility problems became more evident)

MRI Scanning

ost people have an MRI scan (magnetic resonance imaging) during the diagnostic process to identify areas of damage, or lesions, in the brain or spinal cord.

Evoked Potentials

These are simple electrical tests, carried out on vision, hearing or sensation, which can detect a delay in messages from the eyes, ears or skin reaching the brain.

Lumbar Puncture

A sample of fluid is sometimes drawn off from around the spine and tested for signs, which can indicate MS. This test is less routinely used nowadays.

TYPES OF MS

MS is often divided into four different types:

1 Benign

Very occasional relapses, with complete recovery - or remission - in between and no significant disability. Some neurologists put the number of people with benign MS who are leading "normal" lives at higher than 20%.

2 Relapsing/remitting

At diagnosis, about two thirds of people have this form of MS - relapses (or attacks, or exacerbations) on average once or twice per year, with good or complete remission in between, but with a tendency for symptoms to worsen very gradually over time.

3   Secondary Progressive

Some people who begin with relapsing/remitting MS convert after a period of years to this form, in which the severity and frequency of the relapses decrease but disability slowly increases.

4   Primary Progressive

About 10% of people experience, from onset, symptoms that become progressively worse over a period of years without remission.

What is a relapse?

A sudden worsening of symptoms lasting anything from a few days to a few months.   Many people ask if there is any way of reducing the risk of relapse. Unfortunately relapses are unpredictable and there is very little that can be done to stop a relapse once it starts, or reduce the number and severity of relapses. For some people, increased body temperature, due to too hot a bath, hot climate or perhaps an infection, can worsen symptoms and occasionally even cause a relapse.

There is some evidence that stressful life events, such as a car accident or severe emotional stress, can make a relapse more likely. I have found that when suffering an illness all your effort and concentration is channelled on you becoming better. The endeavour however is exasperated when the illness you suffer is life long, and the prognosis is unknown. This can and in some cases will bring on a state of depression as you begin thinking on the negative side of your life and what the future will hold. The stress brought on by this state of mind is more difficult to reduce and you will need your friends with the so called kick up the arse, to put you on the first step to reducing it. Its hard, its bloody hard, to remove the black shroud which you think is surrounding you, but when its gone, your life can move on.

Trying to eliminate daily stressful events and living or trying to live a relaxing lifestyle, without worrying over trivial matters such as housework etc, can reduce the risk of a relapse. However even this is controversial and in any case such stresses are usually unavoidable. (BUT TRY IF YOU CAN and listen to what your body is telling you)

My relapses have been due to family stress and not listening to what my body is telling me(in other words, a cocky bastard). Then its time to be sent to hospital by my GP and undergo a three day course of intravenous steroids, which brings me back to reality. This is my kick start for another twelve to eighteen months, depending on my life events.

My Stress Reduction System (try and let life cut you some slack)

* Don't try to be perfect, YOUR NOT. (I thought I was)
* Learn to say NO, repeatedly. (hard to do sometimes)
* Switch off and do nothing regularly (I am a master at this)
* Don't ever feel guilty (I don't)
* Schedule time just for yourself
* Don't be a martyr and spread yourself too thin
* At times, be untidy and a slob
* Be your own best friend

Predicting the future.......

Although some early symptoms, such as those associated with sight and sensations, often indicate a good prognosis or disease course; it is impossible to say with any certainty how each person's MS will develop.

'One person described his symptoms as his mind was slowly divorcing his body, as he was gradually finding it difficult to control some of his movements.'

> *Please don't say, How are you today,*
> *The answer may be more than I can say,*
> *You may hear a lot more than you wish to hear*
> *So be prepared for the language of fear.*

3 LIVING WITH MS

I am always such pain
I often take the lords name in vain
Can't see an end to my problems as yet
The solution I am awaiting, I have still to get

NO TWO PEOPLE WITH MS experience the same symptoms to the same degree. Most people with MS only experience a few symptoms. Some symptoms are very responsive to treatment; others unfortunately are not.

Because of the diversity of symptoms, treatment is best handled by a multi-disciplinary team of health professionals which may include, for example, a doctor, nurse, physiotherapist, occupational therapist and complementary therapists. With proper symptom management, people should rarely need to be treated for MS in hospital, unless you over do it and wreck yourself.

Some of the more common symptoms are listed below, with an indication of how they can be treated or managed. If you are experiencing these symptoms and need help, ask your GP to help you access specialists. Don't suffer in silence!

Bladder and bowel problems

Bladder problems often include both frequency and urgency and the most common bowel problem is constipation, (probably due to poor diet and a sedentary lifestyle). Although these symptoms are obviously amongst the most distressing, they are also amongst the most responsive to treatment. Specialist continence advice (which can be accessible without your GP) is therefore essential, especially if you are needing to urinate very frequently. Timing your intake of fluids can help, for example, and medications may also be effective for this type of bladder dysfunction. Some people make the mistake of drinking less liquid to cut down on visits to the toilet, but this can actually make problems worse. Low amounts of concentrated urine encourage infection and irritate the bladder. Low fluid intake can also cause constipation. Many people have reported improvements in their bladder and bowel control, after a prolonged course of hyperbaric oxygen therapy.

There are many aids and appliances available, for men and women, to help manage leaks and accidents. These include catheters (thin tubes that help to empty the bladder); sheaths for men; and different types of pads and pants, disposable and washable. You may need more than one kind of product, for example one for during the day and another for at night. To find out what would be best for you, you can contact a specialist continence adviser. You don't need a referral from your GP and most people get an appointment fairly quickly.

Fatigue

Perhaps the commonest MS symptom, this overwhelming sense of exhaustion and weariness can be helped by time management and energy conservation techniques, pacing oneself and by alternating periods of activity with periods of rest. It can be best described as having a small amount of energy per day and when it is used up; you must stop and rest to charge your energy up again. An occupational therapist and physiotherapist is trained to advise on the best ways to manage fatigue. A combination of hyperbaric oxygen and complementary therapies can be an immense fatigue buster as well as resting and listening to relaxation music, which in itself de-stresses the body. Being exhausted may bring on a relapse, so listen to your body; it knows what is best for itself.

Steps for sustaining energy

*   Always have breakfast, no matter how little.

*   Drink plenty of clean (i.e. filtered or bottled) water – ideally, at least 1.5 to 2 litres a day.

*   Eat at least five portions of fresh fruit and vegetables a day.

* Eat at least three meals a week using vegetable sources of protein.

* Eat complex carbohydrates such as wholemeal pasta rather than refined simple carbohydrates such as biscuits, sweets and white bread.

* Avoid stimulants such as coffee, tea, alcohol and nicotine (tobacco.)

* Always chew your food well and try not to eat in a hurry.

* Never over-eat.

Note: Eating in a hurry and over-eating can slow you down more than anything else.

Mobility

Difficulties with walking can be caused by balance or co-ordination problems, dizziness, muscle weakness and spasticity in the joints. This really is a case for a multi-disciplinary management approach, which incorporating gentle exercise can be of benefit. (use it or loose it) For me, keeping cool helps and it means that I can do more throughout the day.

Pain

Pain in MS may be neurological (due to nerve damage) and can include stabbing pains, extreme skin sensitivity and burning sensations or musculoskeletal (due to damage to the tendons, ligaments, muscles and bones.) To treat pain effectively - and for many people it can be treated - the cause of the pain must be identified. Dealing with neurological pain may involve the use of drugs whereas musculoskeletal pain is best treated on the advice of a physiotherapist and/or occupational therapist since it often needs correction of bad posture and positioning.

Spasm

Nerve damage can increase the sensitivity of muscles and cause them to contract into tight, often painful spasm. Apart from being distressing, if untreated, the functioning of the muscles can be affected. Physiotherapists and doctors both play an important role in the management of spasm often through a combination of exercising and drug therapy.

Tremor

An uncontrolled shaking (usually of the head or neck and sometimes in the hand or arm) is one of the hardest symptoms of MS to deal with. Again, physiotherapists can help with coping strategies and some people respond to drug therapies.

Visual disturbances

Eye problems are often an early MS symptom and can include temporary loss of vision, double vision, eye pain and reduction in colour vision. Corticosteroid drugs are often used to reduce the severity of symptoms. Hyperbaric Oxygen Therapy can also be of help.

Mind and Memory

Apart from those already mentioned, some cases of MS can have a mental dimension, affecting a patients cognitive functions, from memory to decreased concentration as the ability to complete complex tasks becomes more difficult. Not everyone with MS experiences cognitive impairment and for those who do, the effects are usually very subtle in the beginning.

> *Please don't tell me you know how I feel.*
> *No one knows how anyone else really feels.*
> *Two people with the same disease will feel totally different*
> *and you are not a bloody mind reader.*

30

4 DRUG THERAPIES

What on earth can I do now
Just sit, wait and wonder how
MS is here but for how long?
They say cure is still yet to be found

There are three kinds of drug therapies used to treat MS:

1) Drugs to manage particular symptoms - Such as spasm, pain or bladder problems.

2) Drugs which treat acute attacks or relapses - Corticosteroids, often referred to simply as steroids, are sometimes given to speed up recovery from a relapse. They can be given either as tablets, intravenous drip or by injection over a short period.

3) Drugs, which modify the disease course - Previously, treatments for MS have been directed at managing symptoms. The last several years, however, have seen the licensing of drugs that can affect the course of MS itself – the disease modifying drugs.

In MS, the body's own immune system appears to start attacking myelin, the protective coating around nerve fibres in the central nervous system, and these disease modifying drugs are thought to suppress the immune response in MS against myelin, although not a cure for MS. The disease modifying drugs for multiple sclerosis licensed in the UK are beta interferon (two kinds: 1a and 1b) and glatiramer acetate. The license confirms that the drugs are effective and safe to the extent claimed by the manufacturers and allows pharmaceutical companies to market them in the UK.

The trade names for beta interferon 1a are Avonex and Rebif. Beta interferon 1b has the trade name Betaferon. The trade name for glatiramer acetate is copaxone.

Who can benefit?

People with relapsing remitting MS: In clinical trials, the beta interferons and glatiramer acetate have reduced relapse rate by approximately one third over a two-year period. The beta interferons also appear to have some impact on the progression of disability.

People with secondary progressive MS: Beta interferon 1b (Betaferon) is the only drug licensed for the treatment of secondary progressive MS. The other drugs have not proved beneficial. Clinical trials have shown some benefit to people with secondary progressive MS but only where relapses are the cause of increasing disability. The drug is not known to benefit people who are already severely disabled.

People with primary progressive MS: There is currently no evidence showing clinical benefits of these drugs for people with primary progressive MS. Research continues in this area. For example, the 'PROMISE' trial, an advanced clinical trial, is assessing the effectiveness of glatiramer acetate for the treatment of primary progressive MS.

Medications that can Relieve MS Symptoms

Stiffness/Spasticity: Baclofen (Lioresal) is an excellent medication for muscle spasms. It can be taken several times per day, and adjusted for those times when your symptoms are at their worst. It can cause some sedation, as well as muscle weakness, since it acts to relax the muscles. For this reason, it must be started at a low dose and increased in small, incremental doses up to the lowest dose that relieves the symptoms. If baclofen does not prove to be effective enough, another medication can be used alone, or in conjunction with baclofen. A newer medication, called tizanidine (Zanaflex) is quite potent, and must be started at a low dose, and increased slowly, as it is very effective in controlling spasms, but is more likely to cause weakness. Finally, a third drug called dantrolene (Dantrium) is sometimes used if the other medications are not effective enough.

Neuropathic pain: There are numerous medications that can be used to trace the pain syndromes that MS causes. There are many medications that are narcotics nor habit-forming that can help to alleviate the pain in the long-term. These include anti-epileptic drugs such as gabapentin (Neurontin), anti-depressants such as amitriptyline (Elavil) and the newer anti-depressants such as sertraline (Zoloft) and paroxetine (Paxil). Although these were traditionally used to treat depression, they have also been found to work in chronic pain syndromes.

Fatigue: Amantidine (Symmetrel) is a medication that can be used to treat sensation of generalized fatigue in MS. It does not work in the muscle fatigue as it occurs with over-exertion, but rather, in the feeling of sleepiness that occurs in MS. Modafinil (Provigil) is a drug used in the treatment of narcolepsy and has also been effective in relieving MS fatigue in patients, at 200mg daily.

Bladder symptoms: Oxybutynin (Ditropan) and tolterodine (Detrol) are medications that can be used to diminish the sensation of urinary urgency and frequency that often occurs as a result of MS.

As I have said and will keep on saying, there is no miracle cure, so drugs / medication may work for one but not another, try you must but don't be disappointed. I have tried so many drugs and treatments, even to having my bloody arm stabbed with B12 injections once a week and am still looking for some respite.

At present I am taking fluroxatine which is an anti depressant and a mixture of cod liver oil and evening primrose oil, they make me feel better about myself and help with relaxation. So with all the above mentioned drugs, I've been there and got numerous tee shirts and I am not letting disappointment drag me down. You have to try because I believe its out there somewhere.

The following two paragraphs have been taken from the Internet and show the groundbreaking progress now being taken in the USA:

www.sciencedaily.com   www.newswise.com

INITIAL CHEMOTHERAPY TREATMENT
REDUCES RELAPSES IN MS PATIENTS

Mitoxantrone, a chemical routinely used to fight breast cancer, leukaemia and malignant lymphoma, has found a new disease to battle: Multiple Sclerosis. Used in an initial intensive course of chemotherapy (induction therapy), mitoxantrone dramatically decreases disease activity in MS patients for at least four years, according to a study presented at the Annual Meeting of the American Academy of Neurology.

Induction therapy, frequently used against cancers, is designed to wipe out abnormal cells and allow for the regrowth of normal cells. The U.S. Food and Drug Administration have recently approved Mitoxantrone for the treatment of MS. It has been used to treat MS in France for more than a decade. Researchers from CHU Pontchaillou of Rennes, France, have demonstrated that mitoxantrone induction therapy for relapsing-remitting MS patients has produced dramatic results in disease activity.

Over the past ten years, 100 worsening relapsing-remitting MS patients were given initial mitoxantrone induction therapy for six months, with mitoxantrone combined with methylprednisolone administered intravenously on a monthly schedule. The annual relapse rate decreased significantly from 3.20 during the 12 months preceding mitoxantrone onset to 0.30 during the first year following induction onset, corresponding to a reduction of nearly 90 percent that was maintained for more than five years. The percentage of relapse-free patients was 76 percent at one year of follow-up, and was maintained at 64 percent, 45 percent, and 43 percent at years two, three and four, respectively, with a median time to the first relapse of 2.8 years.

"The clinical benefit and reduction of disease activity supports our belief that mitoxantrone, as administered in this study, may be an effective induction treatment before initiating other long-term studies.

SECOND PATIENT WITH MULTIPLE SCLEROSIS
UNDERGOES GROUNDBREAKING SURGERY AT YALE

New Haven, Conn. – A 29 year old man with Multiple Sclerosis is the second patient to undergo transplantation surgery at Yale in an effort to repair myelin, the protective brain and spinal cord sheath that is destroyed by the disease, Yale researchers have reported. The surgery took place in two stages March 6-7 2002 and the patient was discharged from Yale-New Haven Hospital March 10 2002. The young man is the second of five patients who are scheduled to participate in the groundbreaking clinical trial.

"The patient is doing fine," said Timothy Vollmer, M.D., associate professor of neurology at Yale School of Medicine. "He has a high level of disability because of the location of the lesions in the brain, but he is otherwise healthy."

There are an estimated 2.4 million persons worldwide with Multiple Sclerosis. The young man in the trial suffers from a relapsing form of Multiple Sclerosis, which Vollmer said is the most common form of Multiple Sclerosis. It affects three times as many women as men.

The purpose of the Phase One trial is to determine whether cells found in the body's peripheral nerves, in this case, the ankle, can safely repair the damaged cells in the brain and spinal cord that result in neurologic disability in patients with Multiple Sclerosis and other disorders of myelin. In Multiple Sclerosis, the immune system attacks the brain's nerve fibers and strips away the protective myelin sheath around nerve fibers in the spinal cord and brain. The resulting lesions make it difficult for the nerves to transmit messages.

In the first procedure on March 6, the surgical team harvested Schwann cells survive in the brain and if they are able to restore myelin on the nerve fibers in the brain. The patient's progress is then monitored for six months using neuroimaging and other tests. After six months a small biopsy is taken to determine whether the cells survived and whether they made any myelin.

The six-month results on the first patient will not be made public until they are published in a peer-reviewed medical journal.

STEM CELL RESEARCH AND THARAPEY

This treatment is probably the most exiting and far reaching to date, but although it seems to be a major step forward, this treatment is still in its infancy. Hailed as possibly the holy grail of medicine, its secrets have yet to be realised to their full potential.

Stem cells are the elemental cells in the body. The first stem cells start in a developing embryo. It is understood that these stem cells are capable of differentiating into every cell type in the human body. Many of the incurable diseases like MS are a result of degeneration of cell types in the body, so by the introduction of healthy new stem cells into the body, the repair and replacement of lost or damaged cells is now hope for the immediate future.

As I have said, this is still in its infancy and at present not available in this country. The cases in the press and news coverage are from people who have travelled to Holland or Belgium and to coin a phrase, "the jury is still out" as to a marked success.

The cost of such treatment is roughly £12,000.00, with differing success rates from the individuals who have undergone the treatment. Of all the who tries what and it works for me therapy's, this one really doe's sound like the one to put your money on, as it sounds so bloody logical its likely to work.

I am not going to drone on about stem cell this and that, as this book is the goal posts for you to find your goal but the following web sites will offer you more of what you may be looking for.

www.stem-cells.com   or   www.cells4health.com

I have been in contact with the stem cell website and have had a consultation with their doctor in America. To date I have not carried this any further, although I was excepted onto their programme, I still feel that there is further research to be done in this field.

*Please don't tell me about your Aunt Doreen,
her MS and how she's managing in spite
of it. I am definitely not your Aunt Doreen
and I am trying to do my best.*

5 Oxygen Therapy

Trying oxygen therapy is a must
It can restore your energy and wonder lust
But you must commit, just give it a go
Just be prepared that progress can be a little slow

OXYGEN-O2
HYPERBARIC OXYGEN THERAPY

Hyperbaric oxygen (HBO) is oxygen at an increased level of pressure. Under increased pressure there is a higher concentration of oxygen coming into contact with any saturating tissue and blood. All the cells in the body are bathed in this oxygen. Hyperbaric Oxygen Therapy is used to treat over 40 types of illness and injury. The theory behind the benefits of hyperbaric oxygen to Multiple Sclerosis lies in fighting the effects of fatty blockages found in the tiny blood vessels of an MS patient. Dr. Philip James, MS Action's Hyperbaric specialist, believes that fat embolism, blockage of fat globules, is responsible for the damage to blood vessels at the onset of every new MS symptom. The damaged vessels leak toxic substances into the surrounding nerve tissues, damaging the myelin sheaths and producing the scattered scars of multiple sclerosis in the central nerve system. HBO treatment works because oxygen, when breathed under pressure, dislodges the fat globules and disperses them. Pressure is the crucial part of delivering oxygen in sufficient quantity to the body, using oxygen at an increased atmospheric pressure reduces the diameter of blood vessels in the nervous system. Despite the reduction in blood-flow, the delivery of oxygen to the tissues is in fact increased. This may sound like a paradox, but it's true. The aim of oxygen treatment in MS is thus to minimize the amount of damaged caused, promote rapid healing and limit scar formation, which can prevent nerve function being restored.

Hyperbaric oxygen therapy is not a cure for MS-whilst many people report improvement in their symptoms (especially for bladder, vision and fatigue problems) or that HBO has helped stabilize their MS. To gain any benefits from HBO, a commitment is required from the patient. When treatment begins 20 sessions, if possible one each day, over consecutive days must be completed. During this time through filling out evaluation sheets, an optimal depth will be established; this will either be at 8, 16, 24 or 33 feet. After the initial 'kick start' it is necessary to 'top up' approximately once a week indefinitely.

A typical MS Hyperbaric chamber looks like a big capsule; it can seat up to six people and has four portholes. Each seat is equipped with an oxygen supply to which a mask will be connected. During treatment (sometimes called a 'dive'-even though there is no water involved in the process) the oxygen mask is worn over the mouth and nose to breathe pure oxygen. The chamber is brought to depth; by the operator who will communicate to you through an intercom (there is a video camera as well to monitor the chamber.) As the session starts the pressure will slowly increase, similar to that of an airplane and patients will feel a slight pressure in their ears (it is the only part of the treatment that could be called unpleasant, and swallowing is the easy solution to equalize the pressure.) Once the chamber has reached depth (it doesn't actually move or go anywhere-it's just that the atmosphere in the chamber has changed to that of one found in the sea) patients will stay at that atmosphere, breathing pure oxygen for one hour (please note, breathing oxygen feels no different than breathing normal air.) After this hour is up, the operator will slowly bring it 'up' to normal atmospheric pressure, the air lock door will open and the session is finished.

There are over 60 Ms Therapy centres and support groups throughout the United Kingdom, 56 of which operate their own Hyperbaric Oxygen Therapy chambers.

Tips for an enjoyable HBO session

* Avoid the temptation to have a cup of tea or coffee before the dive as the door is air locked and there is not a loo in the chamber, it takes a bit of time to bring the chamber back to normal atmospheric pressure.

* Wear comfortable clothing (no nylon or static prone materials please) you may want to bring a blanket in with you as the temperature drops, as the chamber is being re-pressurised.

* Do not take cigarettes, lighters, matches, cellular phones and battery operated car central locking devices in the chamber with you for safety reasons. It may be advisable not to wear your watch in the chamber, as it may not stand up to the pressure.

* Do not use the chamber if you feel a cold or flu coming on, as oxygen will fuel the virus.

* Bring a good book or a magazine in the chamber with you. Chess, dominoes and the (quiet) like can also be played in the chamber.

Comments by HBO patents

I felt a bit tired after the first few sessions of HBO but a few weeks on I was able to clean my house from top to bottom-something I haven't been able to do in over two years.

I can't quite explain how HBO works, and it's not as though I feel an immediate improvement after the session, but if for some reason I miss my weekly top up dive I find myself very tired, and know I need a dive.

I had double vision for nearly a year before I tried HBO, since starting HBO five years ago the double vision has never returned.

I have tried a full course of HBO therapy, which seemed to work but the benefits were short lived (about 3 Hours) I studied my condition and came up with an answer. It was not the HBO which made me feel better but the hours rest in the cold which was more beneficial to my condition.

The following conditions have also been treated with Hyperbaric Oxygen Therapy, giving some measure of success.

Angina, Arthritis, Asphyxiation, Asthma, Carbon Monoxide Poisoning, Cerebral Palsy, Closed Head Injury, Cluster Headache, Collapsed Eardrum, Cystoid Macular Oedema, Diabetes, Enchephalitis, Epilepsy, Frostbite, Gingivitis, Hepatitis C, Hydrocephalus, Leg Ulcers, ME-chronic fatigue syndrome, Meniere's Syndrome, Migraines, Heart Attack, Open Fractures, Osteoarthritis, Perforated Eardrum, Pernicious Anaemia, Radiation Damage, Reye's Syndrome, Sciatica, Shoulder Injury, Sinus Conditions, Spastic Quadrapelia following E-Coli Meningitis, Stroke, Suppurating Abscess, Von Willebrand's Disease.

Liquid Health, is this a new science? Aerobic Oxygen/Hydroxygen

A revolutionary new break-through helps eliminate tiredness, provide energy, vitality and alertness, by introducing more oxygen into the body.

The evidence seems overwhelming. Oxygen plays a powerful primary role in our health and well being. The more oxygen we have in our system, the more energy we produce. Understanding this is more important than ever before, because of a general deficiency of oxygen intake. Simply put, the best way to optimize health is to be sure that we oxygenate every cell in our body. (Dr Norman McVea)

It's true that energy is primarily a function of oxygen. Unless you have sufficient oxygen in your body, everything about you can be affected. Your physical capacity to work effectively, your energy and vitality are drained.

New Science?

Oxygen therapy has been used for decades to treat the sick, for example oxygen tents and masks, etc. but over the last 50 years scientists around the world have continually tried to harness the powerful health enhancing properties of oxygen for use in the body other than breathing. No formulation has been successful until the invention of Aerobic Oxygen or Hydroxygen Plus

This breakthrough discovery – the process of stabilizing high concentrates of oxygen molecules in a non-toxic liquid form, has revolutionized oxygen therapy around the world.

The Hidden Secret?

Aerobic Oxygen/ Hydroxygen Plus, contains negatively charged electrons that have attached themselves to molecules of oxygen thus creating ionized oxygen. You are already familiar with ionized oxygen if you've smelled the air after a thunderstorm. You feel great, revitalized and alert. The lightening from the storm adds a small negatively charged electron to each oxygen molecule in a process called ionization.

Ionized oxygen in liquid form has positive advantages when taken internally. It has an effect very similar to pure oxygen. It is more readily absorbed by your system. The more of these negatively charged molecules of oxygen that enter your body the healthier you feel. They energize your brain and make you feel more alive and alert. Research indicates that taking oxygen supplements assist the body in improving vitamin, mineral and nutritional absorption along with increasing energy and enhancing the immune system.

But there is a but, a big but, because there is no or very little profit in oxygen, the drug company's with their billions don't push research into this branch of medicine. Life seems to be in the hands of the $ and £ I am sorry to say.

My walking gait's like I am a drunken man,
Please don't judge me, as I am what I am,
I try my best to keep upright,
While most of the time I feel like shite.

6 Relationships & Sexual Health

Why Am I affected, why did it happen to me?
When it comes to sex, no problem I see
I love the warmth, the glow and touch
Oh, I really love sharing sex so much

WHEN ONE PERSON in the family has MS, then it effects the whole family unit.   Be prepared for a rough ride as depression, anger, anxiety and the biggest dose of the fuckems you are ever likely to get tries to take a hold. This is because the simplest of every day living tasks become difficult as the disease tries to dictate your future and you become a bastard to live with some of the time. For you, the love for your partner is not in question, so try some reassurance, its not there fault you have become the monster with two heads. (I know as I am speaking from experience)

If or when its time you think you may need carers to come and take some of the burden off your partner, DO IT. Your partner is your partner not your nurse, never mind in sickness and in health, that's bullshit. If you want your relationship to continue, cut them some slack and let others do some of the work, let them be your loving partner, they need love as well as you.

A strong and loving relationship with ones partner, I believe is as equally as much to do with facing and fighting the condition as everything else. To have the support and reassurance of a loved one in the fight ahead, is of up most importance, as many relationships have broken down due to the future looking grim as disability takes a hold. (It happened to me after 29 years of marriage). But what about me, I am handsome, funny and a new love I am confident I will find. I had MS for fifteen years and as my mobility deteriorated I had to give up work and live on benefits and a works pension. The old saying of when poverty comes through the door love goes out of the window was true in my case. But the lord works in mysterious ways!!! 4 weeks after my wife deserted me for someone else who could walk and left me supposedly on the scrap heap, I met someone else. The new love I have is stronger, accepting of my condition and now sex is unconditional and meaningful)

Problems resulting from MS that are not really specific to any one particular part of the body – though sexual problems clearly involve mainly the sexual organs and do not necessarily have direct physical causes. For example, a sexual problem such as impotence is obviously a physical symptom but it can just as easily be the result of feeling fatigued and depressed at having MS. In that sense it is not at all specific to people with MS. Impotence is a problem common to many men.

Sexual problems of tiredness and depression are thought to be separate; in reality they are closely linked. Depression can lead to tiredness that can lead to sexual problems, and sexual problems can lead to depression that can lead to tiredness, and so on.

But though it is true that mental and emotional problems that anyone can experience can cause sexual problems – it can also be caused by work or money problems. It is also true that sexual problems in MS can be the result of causes that are specific to MS.

Meeting and falling in love with someone with MS, is not all doom and gloom

A true encounter:-

I must say from the onset, I was not looking for any romantic relationship. I had just come out of a 23-year marriage and was emotionally abused, but perhaps that is when you are most likely to meet someone.

From the beginning I was aware that he had MS and used a wheelchair, but that did not matter to me. It began just as a friendship and if I am honest, it would not have begun as a relationship partly through my own lacking of self-confidence and also through my perception of someone who used a wheelchair. I was under the impression that the act of making love was totally out of the question.

I got to know a very special, sensitive and kind person through a strong friendship which developed into a very deep love, one which is not only sexually fulfilling but is also on an equal footing. Everything is shared and halved and one key to all this is communication and alternatives. If he is ill and cannot do things he explains how he feels so there is no wrong assumptions being made and if possible alternatives can be compromised. For example we may have made arrangements with friends to go out for a meal and he is so tired it would not be possible for him. We would invite the friends round and order a Chinese or something. That way he does not feel that he is letting me down in someway.

My children were 12 and 10 when they met him. My daughter of 12 would not offer to push the wheelchair when we were out and I wrongly thought is was because she was embarrassed, when the real reason was that she was frightened of hurting him or tipping him out. They have since learned to accept him, which is easy with his easy going sense of humour and now fight for who is to push him. They sometime forget and argue with him which I am sure makes him feel more "normal" in everyday life.

The life I now have is different I do not know what the future will bring, but who does? I only know I live happily in a loving relationship with my daughters and the man I love.

The forthright account of a partner

Physical causes of sexual problems in women with MS are commonly lack of vaginal lubrication and sensation, muscle spasm and poor bladder control coupled with decreased ability to have an orgasm, while in men the problem is mainly an inability to have an erection (impotence) or ejaculate also leading to reduced orgasm experience.

Drugs given for MS can also be to blame. Some tranquillisers and antidepressants can depress sexual response, as can tobacco, cannabis, cocaine and too much alcohol. Other physical causes of what doctors call sexual 'dysfunction', particularly of impotence in men, is heart disease, diabetes, having mumps as an adult and anti-ulcer drugs.

Having MS is no reason whatsoever to stop or limit sexual activity if you don't want to and fortunately, a wide variety of treatments is available that can be very effective for both men and women in helping to maintain both the desire and the means. Covering psychological as well as physical needs, these include counselling and psychotherapy, massage with aromatherapy oils, reflexology, nutritional therapy (diet and supplements) and exercise.

General treatments for lack of sexual desire and impotence

Whatever the underlying reasons for the problem you are experiencing the first need for anyone worried about reduced sexual response is to talk about it. Talking about it – communicating your anxieties and concerns – is very definitely the first step to solving it. Obviously your partner is the best person to talk to if you can, since he or she is the person most affected and the closest to you.

If this is not possible for any reason, as sexual problems are often some of the hardest for couples to share, then my advice, like I did, was to talk to my doctor. (We talked about the problems I was having and the effect it seemed to be putting on the relationship with my partner, but in the end my problems were nothing to do with my MS) Of course if you are confident in your doctor then there is no problem. And sometimes you may well need the advice of someone with specialist medical knowledge.

Most of the time a doctor will probably refer you to a trained counsellor, psychotherapist or even sex therapist anyway and seeing a specialist in listening to problems and suggesting solutions is also an excellent option, especially one experienced in the sex problems of people with MS.

Since stress and anxiety can be one of the biggest causes of sexual problems this one step alone can work wonders as it can help to remove the underlying tension they can produce. Many therapists won't just stop at talking though. They are quite likely to suggest other approaches to help you relax and feel more at peace with yourself as well as, at the same time, reawaken your needs and desires.

Good advice for anyone, man or woman, wanting to improve their sexual health is:

* Eat a good balanced diet
* Do regular exercise
* Cut out smoking
* Don't drink too much alcohol

In addition I would recommend the following, particularly for those with MS:

* Massage with essential oils (aromatherapy)
* Reflexology

Nutritional therapy - Diet and nutrition

Diet and exercise are two of the most effective ways of stimulating your body to respond sexually, mainly because they are both vital for overall health and vitality, and in an adult a healthy and vital body is a sexual body. So make sure you not only keep active by exercising but by eating properly. That means not only eating a balanced diet but, for sexual problems, foods that are good for the sexual or reproductive system.

Fortunately foods that are good for the reproductive system in adults are also very tasty so there is no real excuse for avoiding this part of the programme. In fact most people find it very enjoyable! For example, three of the most important nutrients for the reproductive system are the vitamins C and E and the mineral zinc (particularly important for men.)

Please don't decide what I am capable of doing.
Allow me to decide what activities I can do.
There may be times I might make the wrong
Decision and if I do, I'll know it soon enough.

Food supplements for sexual health

Nutrient	Daily dose	Action
MEN		
Zinc	15mg	Supports prostate gland and sex organs
Vitamin C	1000mg	Improves sperm quality and mobility
Vitamin E	400iu	Increases fertility and restores potency
L-Arginine	500mg	Increases sperm count
WOMEN		
Zinc	15mg	Supports reproductive organs
Vitamin C	1000mg	Supports repair and growth of tissue cells
Vitamin E	400iu	Increases fertility and strengthens cells.

7 Rehabilitation

Rehabilitation became my new friend
Ideas on exercise they did send
The increase in energy made me feel good and well
After a short while everyone could tell

HOW CAN REHABILITATION HELP, when MS progresses? Rehabilitation for people with MS can help at all stages, from diagnosis onwards. It can help to modify the more troublesome effects of some MS symptoms and help people to stay as independent as possible.

At its heart is a holistic approach; an understanding that a person's needs must be addressed at different levels, medical, environmental, social, and personal, because all these aspects of experience have an effect on a person's quality of life.

Rehabilitation includes helping people to make the most of their physical capabilities, by maintaining physical function, for example, by teaching new techniques for daily living, and by adaptations to people's environments. It includes emotional support, from enabling people to adjust, physically and psychologically, in 'helping people find a reason to get up in the morning'.

Given the complexity of MS and the difficulties that arise from it, the involvement of a range of specialists is essential. No single specialist can provide all the care a person needs and research evidence has highlighted the need for different professionals to be involved, from assessment onwards. 'A multi-disciplinary assessment is the key to rehabilitation.'

PHYSIOTHERAPY

Both research and a wealth of user experience show that physiotherapy has a vital role in containing the effects of MS. The sooner a person diagnosed with Multiple Sclerosis starts physiotherapy the better the

48

prognosis for the future. Many of the complications of MS arise from misuse and inactivity, not to mention that it is easier to maintain existing use of limbs rather than to try to regain the use of limbs that have become disabled.

Gentle (and I must stress gentle) and routine exercise is the key to improving your mobility and general MS condition. It is no good at all trying to be another Mr universe, when you were not one before. Too much physical strain on the body, especially in the beginning, will have an adverse effect and will most likely bring on a relapse. I know, because I tried to push myself as the benefits to my condition increased due to exercise, but in the end I became ill and had to stop, as I was physically exhausted. Every persons MS is different, but when beginning on an exercise strategy, similar types of exercise are suitable for all and much can be achieved with group sessions, as you can share the experience.

Some of the symptoms of MS, such as muscle weakness or spasm, occur as a secondary symptom of the initial nerve damage, therefore if the body is persuaded to move normally, even if its reflex responses have diminished, the adverse effect that abnormal movement has on muscles will be delayed. Neuro-physiotherapy works on this basis and is the physiotherapy especially designed for Multiple Sclerosis patients.

The objectives of neuro-physiotherapy are:

* To improve and maintain joint mobility
* To improve balance and co-ordination
* To delay muscle spasms
* To maintain general fitness
* To increase energy levels
* To improve circulation and all body functions

Why exercise is so important when you have MS

Increased energy

You may think exercise will make you fatigued, but done properly; it can have the opposite effect. When we exercise we breathe more strongly and our heart rate increases. We automatically take in more oxygen, which is then carried by the blood around the body, oxygenating the tissues and improving energy levels.

Muscle tone & strength

When you have MS you are less active and not usually able to keep your muscles toned through normal day-to-day activity. Unfortunately this then leads to more mobility problems and more fatigue.

Muscle weakness may not be due to neurological damage but to lack of use. You know what they say: "use it or lose it."

But even when muscles have been weakened through neurological damage, working to keep the brain/muscle connection active will help to stimulate the nerve pathways, (the de-tour effect).

Circulation

Exercise boosts the circulation, strengthens and improves heart and lung function, speeds up the metabolism, and assists the body in the cleansing and removal of toxins. The lymphatic system does not have a pump and therefore we need to exercise to help it excrete toxins and waste products.

Psychological Benefits

The feel good factor is what sends us back to the gym, pool or whatever, time after time. We get that wonderful feeling of contentment and well being after a good workout from all those feel good hormones (the endorphins) whizzing round the brain and the extra oxygen gets to all the body's tissues.

Looking Good

Most of us want to look as good as we can and exercise can help achieve that. Better muscle tone, improved skin colour, feeling more alive and energetic. How can the opposite sex resist?

Posture

Exercise strengthens the spinal muscles, the abdominals and gluteals, thus helping to improve posture. This in turn has a positive effect on breathing and lung function. Poor posture is often one of the root causes of low energy. When we hold ourselves better, the internal organs operate more efficiently thus helping to improve all the body's functions.

Digestion

Exercise stimulates digestion and elimination of waste products, enhancing the uptake of nutrients, and passage of waste through the excretory organs. Many forms of exercise help to stimulate the internal organs. Yoga in particular is brilliant for this.

Joints and Skeleton

Exercise helps keeps joints mobile and bones strong. It also strengthens the support system for the skeleton, the muscles. When muscles are stretched and toned we are able to support the bones and skeleton more effectively thus reducing the risk of pain in the bones and joints. If you are able to do weight bearing exercises, this will help protect you against osteoporosis. These including yoga standing postures, rebounding, and cycling.

Sleep and Relaxation

Once you exercise regularly, sleep patterns improve. Exercise produces a natural level of tiredness rather than an unnatural level of fatigue through inactivity. Also the body is able to relax more effectively after exercise as the mind and body quieten and thoughts become calmer. Often poor sleep patterns are the result of overactive thoughts and an under active body.

What exercise?

1. There are three basic kinds of exercise that we all need to do a little of, as often as possible.

Cardiovascular exercise – for the heart and lungs
Includes swimming, cycling, rebounding, exercise bikes or medimotion type exercisers – anything that pushes up the heart rate and is maintained for at least 5-20 mins, 3 times a week.

2. Muscle strengthening exercise
Includes, weight training, physiotherapy, swimming and yoga.

3. Stretching exercises
Helps to lengthen and stretch muscles, improves flexibility, improves posture, helps counteract tightness in muscle groups and can relieve pain caused by lack of mobility. Includes, yoga, shiatsu (assisted stretching) and physiotherapy stretches. These all help to develop longer muscles, less restricted movements, more comfortable posture and body alignment.

Whatever exercise you do, should be:

Suitable to your abilities
Choose something which is compatible with what you can do in terms of strength and mobility. For instance, for many people with MS, walking and aerobics are not suitable because they are too physically draining.

Fun or at least not boring or tedious
Try out one or two forms of exercise to see which you like best. To stick to an exercise regime for any length of time, you need to enjoy it.

Easily accessible
To develop a regular exercise routine, choose something which takes the minimum amount of organization. Don't choose something that takes you hours to get to or prepare for, you just won't keep it up! If you can, exercise at home in a room which is well ventilated, attractive and comfortable, keep your mat and exercise equipment readily to hand. If space allows, keep a small area set aside so that you can get on with your routine whenever you feel the urge.

Non fatiguing
Never exercise to the point of exhaustion (this may bring on a relapse). Build up slowly. This enables your body to gradually build stamina without causing fatigue. Choosing appropriate exercise will go a long way towards eliminating exercise induced fatigue. Avoid getting too hot as heat slows down nerve conduction and makes us feel exhausted.

Set realistic goals
Set goals that inspire and motivate you, yet are achievable. Every journey starts with one small step. Build up strength, stamina, mobility and flexibility, gradually. It is counterproductive to overdo the exercise in the early stages, because if you do, it will make you feel weaker not stronger, more tired not less. Then you will become disillusioned with what you are doing and simply give up!

Do you also need to take nutritional supplements?

I have found out, through experience, once I added a high quality multi-vitamin/mineral supplement to my diet that I was able to step up my exercise programme and strengthen my body through exercise.

Nutrients I find are particularly good for keeping energy levels high are B vitamins, co-enzyme Q10, vitamin C, calcium, magnesium, iron, zinc and chromium.

Please don't be upset that you cannot ease
my problems. It won't do any good for all
of us to be miserable. At times I seem to hold
a monopoly on being miserable.

8   Complementary Therapies

I don't feel like doing an awful lot
Much use of my limbs I have no longer got
I don't feel like moving about anymore
If only I knew, one day I could do more!

CONDUCTIVE EDUCATION

(www.conductive-education.org   www.conductive-education.org)

The National Institute of Conductive Education (NICE) designs and addresses the main issues around rehabilitation for people with MS. Conductive Education is an educational approach to multiple sclerosis, which helps individuals develop the skills and motivation they need to overcome problems of movement and bodily control they encounter in everyday living.

Specialist educators called conductors, work closely with participants enabling them to re-learn skills that have been lost or discover new ways of achieving them.   Many of the participants speak of increased confidence and self-assurance they gain from taking an active part in finding solutions to the problems they face in everyday living.   This renewed confidence in their abilities enables them to lead more active and independent lives.

HOW CAN CONDUCTIVE EDUCATION HELP ME?

You may have recently been diagnosed with Multiple Sclerosis and be very uncertain of what the future holds for you, or you may have had multiple sclerosis for several years and are beginning to lose control of your mobility, furthermore you would like to do something about it.

Whatever stage you are at with the condition, conductive education can help you to maintain and/or increase the range and control of your movement skills.

Particular emphasis is placed on developing:

* Skills to assist in the reduction of spasticity.
* Skills to improve the control of movements.
* Your uses of rhythm to help you fully utilize your movements.
* Breathing techniques to enhance speech, circulation and general well-being.
* Skills to control eye movements.
* Techniques to overcome continence problems.

WHAT CAN I EXPECT TO GAIN?

* Increased confidence in your own abilities.
* Increase your level of independence.
* Improvements in bodily control and mobility.
* A reduction in 'bad' habits.
* Increase in stamina.
* Improved quality of life.

"After the first week I noticed an improvement in my mobility and I seemed to have more energy. I have greater insight now into the techniques involved in basic mobility eg. Moving my hips. (Participant with multiple sclerosis)"

YOGA

So many theories have been put forward about the suitability of exercise in easing the symptoms MS. At one time sufferers were encouraged to work out in the gym to improve strength and boost energy. Subsequent evidence, through patient's inability to show progress, showed such activities were not suitable, so all exercise then became a personal preference, as everyone's MS is particular to that person and a gentle start is now seen as the way forward. Yoga comes under this gentle exercise heading. One definition of yoga is that it is "action in inaction", implying that, although the body is sometimes held in a position for a few seconds or minutes without any apparent movement, many subtle effects occur.

I believe yoga is great for MS, because it improves the functioning of the hypothalamus gland, which governs the autonomic nervous system that becomes impaired by MS. It also encourages blood flow to the brain stem, which is limited in MS sufferers, and it alleviates the painful build-up of lactic acid in the muscles, which comes through lack of exercise.

Yoga teaches you to breathe efficiently. This is particularly relevant to MS as breath is our chief energy source. It also develops the power of your will – an important factor in recovering from the effects of an MS relapse, as it also promotes relaxation and sleep. MS sufferers who do yoga say they feel more alive and energetic, suffer less pain and find their brain works better. The benefits are cumulative

Since the late 1970's, many people with MS have been doing yoga, as it has proved a great benefit. Yoga is a unity of the mental and physical. Done properly it calms the mind and energizes the body. One of the catch 22s of MS is that stress and tension probably play some part in bringing on an attack of MS, but once you have MS, this in itself creates stress and tensions both physically and mentally. The practice of yoga can help alleviate both the physical and mental stresses and tensions.

* Yoga may help the body's own self-healing mechanism and may slow down or even halt the disease process.
* Yoga stills the mind.
* Yoga increases energy and counteracts fatigue.
* Yoga lifts the mood and counteracts depression.
* Yoga has a good effect on the functioning of the endocrine glands, the circulatory and respiratory system, and improves well-being.
* Yoga does not need any special equipment and you can practice it daily at home.

(Daily Express Women-Clare Gardner 26/8/2002)

REFLEXOLOGY

Reflexology takes a holistic approach to healing, treating the whole person, not just the symptoms. When you are ill, your body is a state of 'imbalance' energy pathways are blocked, and this stops your body from functioning effectively. Reflexology aims to restore the body to a state of balance and natural equilibrium. Reflexologists maintain that your feet are 'mirror images' of your body and that each point on your foot corresponds to a specific part of your body. So, in fact by massaging the foot you are, in fact, massaging the whole body. By applying gentle pressure to these tender points, you can release blockages and restore the free flow of energy to the whole body.

ACUPUNCTURE

Acupuncture is a system of healing first recorded in China and Japan around 4,500 years ago. It is based on the belief that health is dependent on the body's motivating energy (called Qi – which exists in equal and opposite quantities, known as Ying and Yang), moving in a smooth and balanced way through a series of channels beneath the skin. When Qi becomes unbalanced ill health results. There are around 500 recognised acupuncture points on the body, though they don't necessarily lie near the part of the body being treated – for example headaches can be treated on points in the feet or hands.

Because Acupuncture is based on this very comprehensive healing system, the acupuncturist sees each patient as a whole and takes into account all the factors affecting the person's energy system. Environment, diet, occupational, etc are all assessed and the acupuncturist will ask about your symptoms and any treatments you have received so far. MS is not treated as one disease, but rather the person suffering from MS is treated according to his or her individual experience of the disease. Once the acupuncturist has gathered enough information, she inserts fine needles into the channels of energy in the appropriate acupuncture point to stimulate the body's healing response and help restore its balance. The needles are left in place for up to 20 minutes, and you may feel a slight tingling, though it doesn't actually hurt. At some sessions the acupuncturist may opt to use a non-invasive treatment such as Reiki.

CHIROPRACTICS

Information from your mind passes through your brain, along your spinal cord and out across the nerves to the cells of your body. Sensation about how your body is responding and functioning passes back the same way. By expressing this information, your nervous system controls, coordinates and gives life to all the cells and structures of your body. If your nervous system becomes irritated by malfunctions or misalignments of joints (subluxations – common to those with Multiple Sclerosis), particularly those of the spine, pelvis or skull, the flow of information is impeded and the result is a decrease in function of your body's cells.

CHIROPODY

The chiropodist can help with a variety of foot care issues such as nail cutting, ingrown toenails, corns, etc. When mobility is limited it can be very difficult or uncomfortable to cut your own nails though it is imperative not to neglect your feet as some types of treatment such as long term steroids used occasionally to treat MS necessitate frequent checks. Remember you only get one pair of feet, so look after them!

AROMATHERAPY

Aromatherapy is a gentle natural and holistic solution for many health problems especially those that cause stress, back pain and muscular aches and pains. During an aromatherapy treatment essential oils are chosen for specific conditions and ailments and are blended into massage oil. The blend is then applied in a relaxing massage. This treatment combines the therapeutic benefits of massage and essential oils. An Aromatherapy session should last approximately 45 minutes. A detailed medical history is taken at the initial session, and information is taken about your present state – tired, anxious. The massage is extremely relaxing and gentle.

COUNSELLING

Could it help you?   What is counseling?

There are many different types of counselling, each with its own theoretical basis. But, in general, counselling is a 'talking treatment', designed to help people who wish to make changes in their lives.

A counsellor won't give you specific advice, or tell you how to behave. Neither will you just sit there while the counsellor talks at you, counselling is an active, not a passive process. The counsellor will help you explore and work through your feelings, some of which you might not be aware of, allowing you to find your own solutions. The aim is progress and change: following counselling, you should feel better equipped to face the future. 'Counselling is like looking into a mirror and seeing yourself in a different way' the counsellor reflects back to you an image which you might not have seen before. It's not an ordinary relationship: it's one in which change and understanding can be facilitated.' Counselling is strictly confidential and sessions usually last between 45 minutes and one hour. Some people only need one appointment, while others benefit from a series of consultations. Depending on the issues which you wish to address, it may take the form of one-to-one counselling, couple counselling or group counselling.

Unlike medicine, counselling is not a science. There's no absolute proof that it works. But a century of anecdotal evidence reveals that many people find it extremely helpful. However, the decision to start the counselling process must be your own. It won't benefit you unless you want to be there and are prepared to work with the counsellor. It can be difficult and, at times, painful. You have to look closely at yourself and face up to things which you may not find comfortable to address, and you have to want to change and take responsibility for yourself.

Telephone counselling can be extremely useful for dealing with distress instantly, but it isn't a substitute for face-to-face counselling. By its nature, its unstructured and brief, allowing little time for discussion or exploration. Counselling is not the same as psychotherapy, although it isn't always easy to draw a line between them and there are different kinds of psychotherapy. Without getting too technical, it is usually a longer process than counselling and looks more deeply into the way a person's mind works. Having MS may trigger emotional difficulties that someone has already had for many years and people who are interested in exploring the ways their minds work, or people who have always worried about their mental health, may choose to seek psychotherapy rather than counselling, if it is available.

9 Diet & Nutrition

I don't feel like anything to eat
This MS has me totally beat
Why bother cooking food anymore
I still remember when I could eat food galore

DIETARY COUNSELLING

NUTRITION has had extremely positive results as a therapy for controlling Multiple Sclerosis. Nutrition is an umbrella word that can describe the food you eat, nutrients in the form of supplements, the efficiency of your body's absorption and digestion, as well as food that you may be tolerant to ('intolerance' is often confused with 'allergic' but are very different as intolerances are reversible.) Dietary counselling can include food sensitivity screening, which is highly recommended before starting any new diet. Nutritional screening checks for intolerant foodstuffs as well as vitamin, mineral and basic digestion status ensuring the best possible gut efficiency and strengthened immune system. When foodstuffs that the digestive system is intolerant to are continually ingested, not only is the immune system weakened, but partially digested foodstuffs are allowed to pass into the circulation, these are known to be neurotoxic (poisonous to nerve tissue) so of especial detriment to MS sufferers. These toxins need to be removed to prevent further inflammation to the central nervous system tissue. The nutritionist will work further to insure good nutrition, efficient absorption, and proper supplementation.

THE BALANCE OF GOOD HEALTH

A well balanced diet can help you maintain a healthy lifestyle, lessen fatigue and minimize the chance of getting infections. It doesn't have to be restrictive, difficult or expensive.

What is a balanced diet?

A balanced diet should give you all the nutrients you need to stay as healthy as possible:

*   Eat three meals at regular intervals each day.

*   Eat a wide variety of foods from each of the recommended groups, in moderate amounts.

*   Replace high fat or sugary foods with low fat/low sugar alternatives.

*   Cut fat off meat.

*   Grill, steam, bake or poach food instead of frying (throw the frying pan away).

*   Eat high fibre foods.

*   Eat five portions of fruit and vegetables each day.

*   Drink 8-10 cups (1-2 litres) of liquid a day, especially water.

Essential food groups

Every day you should try to eat a variety from each of the four food groups detailed below:

Proteins are important for muscle building and energy. You should try to eat at least two to three portions each day. High protein foods are: lean meat, fish, beans and pulses, and dairy products.

Carbohydrates are starchy foods, which provide energy and should form the basis of your diet. They are found in cereal-based and high fibre foods. Fibre helps to maintain healthy digestion and minimize constipation. Good sources of carbohydrates include: wholemeal bread and flour, cereals (wheat, oats, corn, etc), pasta and rice, beans and pulses, potatoes, fresh and dried fruit.

Dairy products are a good source of calcium, protein and vitamins A, D, E and B (especially folic acid and B12), but are high in saturated fats (which raise cholesterol levels) so choose low fat versions where possible. Dairy products include: milk, yoghurt, cheese, and eggs (which should always be well-cooked.)

Fruit and vegetables are an important source of vitamins A, C and E (anti-oxidants), and minerals such as potassium, magnesium and calcium. You should eat five portions of fresh fruit and vegetables each day. Some people may prefer organic produce. Frozen ones are a nutritious alternative. Don't overcook, steam or boil them in as little water as possible to avoid destroying vitamins and minerals.

Fats – good or bad?

Small amount of fat are an important source of energy. There are three types, but they all have the same calorie content:

*   Saturated – associated with raised cholesterol levels. Found mainly in animal products (i.e. dairy products and meat), processed foods, palm and coconut oil. Keep intake to a minimum.

*   Monounsaturated – not as closely linked with higher cholesterol levels as saturated fats. Found mostly in avocados, olive oil, and nuts (e.g. peanuts, hazelnuts, almonds.)

*   Polyunsaturated – essential fatty acids found mainly in vegetable oils and seeds (e.g. sunflower, Soya, safflower, corn and maize), oily fish and fish oils. Try to eat these in preference to other fats.

All fats are high in calories, so if you are overweight you should limit your intake, especially of saturated fat. Use low fat products such as low fat spreads, low fat cheeses, and semi-skimmed or skimmed milk.

NUTRITION FOR MS

You may want to pay particular attention to the following key aspects of what you eat if you have MS, as every person with MS responds differently to a particular diet and it is up to the individual to find what is tolerant or intolerant to them.

Essential fatty acids (EFAs)

Essential fatty acids are polyunsaturated fats, such as linolenic and alpha-linolenic acid. They play an important role in maintaining the central nervous system and the myelin sheath, so although there is no definitive evidence of long-term benefit, it makes sense to ensure a good intake of EFAs if you have MS.

Linoleic acid is found in sunflower, safflower and Soya oils, and margarines such as Flora and Linusit Gold, which have no hydrogenated fat. Alpha-linolenic acid is mainly found in dark green leafy vegetables (e.g. broccoli, green cabbage, spinach, kale, Brussels sprouts, green peppers, parsley and lettuce), Soya and edible linseed oils, oily fish (e.g. tuna, salmon, mackerel, pilchards and sardines) and fish oils.

Supplements rich in EFAs, such as evening primrose, starflower, and wheatgerm oil are available over the counter, but can be expensive.

Vitamins and minerals

Multiple Sclerosis fighting supplements fall into four general groupings.

* Products that oxygenate the body work in conjunction with products for the immune system.

* Supplements that aid in detoxification work in conjunction with free radical scavengers.

* This group consists of products that help relieve Multiple Sclerosis caused pain, reduce inflammation and protect or help repair the myelin sheath.

* And finally, products that help the body repair possible long term Multiple Sclerosis caused damage to organ and hormonal systems.

In no way am I claiming that any of these products will cure Multiple Sclerosis. I don't feel that there is really any such thing as a "cure" for Multiple Sclerosis, or that any one product or combination of products is going to work a miracle on Multiple Sclerosis. While some of the testimonies may sound rather miraculous, but most of the time any improvement is likely to be slow. What these products do is support the body in a way that it is then able to be more efficient to deal with the dysfunctions and other problems that happen within your body when you have Multiple Sclerosis.

The Multiple Sclerosis fighting, immune system enhancing and oxygenating supplements are the place to start, to work on the autoimmune response attacking the body.

Before we get started, here are a few basics. All autoimmune diseases are closely related. With the same underlying causes of over-toxicity, virus, mycoplasma or bacteria infections, and they are similar in how they affect the body. An autoimmune condition may manifest as Multiple Sclerosis in one person, or chronic fatigue in someone else, because of different genetics, or who knows what. So what applies to chronic fatigue, almost always has some bearing on Multiple Sclerosis too.

And finally, it took years to get your immune system to the point where Multiple Sclerosis could develop. While a certain small percentage of people seem to recover quickly from attacks of Multiple Sclerosis or at least initially, most people take considerably longer to show signs of recovery, if ever.

You decide if any of these health-promoting supplements here are worth trying. Commit to using whatever you choose for at least 90 days.

Otherwise you could be short-changing yourself, and perhaps missing out on a chance of improving your health.

Sufficiently oxygenated cells may be able to kill a significant amount of mycoplasma and viruses. It could possibly even take care of these Multiple Sclerosis causing infections on its own. However, your immune system has got to be made stronger and less dysfunctional if you wish to successful combat Multiple Sclerosis. As even the high-powered antibiotics can't completely kill off the mycoplasmas, you have got to get your immune system back in shape to successfully deal with these infections

Vitamins and minerals

You may not need to take special vitamin supplements if you eat a healthy and varied diet. However, certain vitamins, such as folic acid and B12, are important for a healthy nervous system, so make sure you have a good intake of these in your diet.

Vitamins are easily destroyed by storage and cooking, so eat fresh fruit and vegetables as soon as possible and don't over-cook them.

Good sources of folic acid include: liver, leafy green vegetables, high fibre breakfast cereals (fortified with B12 and folate), beans, pulses and nuts, and dairy products.

Vitamin B12 is only found in animal-based foods. Good sources are liver, beef, kidneys, eggs, milk and cheese. This important vitamin is often deficient in people with MS as it is in vegans (and so a vegan with MS is particularly at risk.) Taking B12 as a supplement is one solution. The right dose is 100mcg a day – although any B vitamin should only be taken as a complex: that is, with all B vitamins together in one capsule.

The importance of vitamin B12 in MS

Vitamin B12 is one of the most important nutrients in MS because B12 is vital to the healthy growth and repair of nerves. Severe B12 deficiency can cause permanent damage to the nervous system. Symptoms of B12 deficiency can take up to five years to show after the body's reserves had been used up.

Symptoms of B12 deficiency are tingling or numbness in the hands and feet, pain in the ends of the fingers and toes, problems with balance, memory and concentration, mental confusion and depression, exhaustion, shortness of breath, problems with mucuous membranes, and anaemia. (Anaemia is caused by iron deficiency but because B12 helps to 'release' iron a B12 deficiency may be the real underlying reason.)

Other people likely to be B12 deficient are those from a family with an inherited tendency to pernicious anaemia, and those from families in which blue eyes and premature greying are common.

Certain drugs can also affect levels of B12 in the body. For example, prolonged use of antibiotics, some anti-diabetic drugs, the cholesterol-lowering agent cholestyromine, and potassium chloride supplements can all reduce levels of B12 and create a deficiency.

The trouble with B12 if you have MS, though, is that it is not really enough to take a capsule or the right food. According to research, one of the features of MS is a lack of the right digestive enzymes and so people with MS often have difficulty absorbing B12 in the normal way through the stomach wall. That's why B12 is usually given to people with MS by injection: the stomach is by-passed and the vitamin goes straight into the blood supply where it is needed. Injection is normally done by a medical doctor.

Antioxidants

Betacarotene and vitamins A, C and E are antioxidants which help to minimize the risk of heart disease and some cancers, as well as maintaining a healthy nervous system. To ensure you are getting enough of these vitamins you should eat at least five portions of fruit and vegetables daily. If you are concerned about your intake of vitamins and minerals, talk to your doctor or ask to be referred to a dietitian.

Is there a special diet for MS?

Claims have been made for many diets said to help MS – low fat, gluten-free, dairy-free, etc. So far, no controlled studies have been carried out, so there is no conclusive scientific evidence of any being beneficial, as everyone with MS reacts differently to a particular diet. Some diets can be very restrictive and expensive. They may be bad for your health if followed without supervision by your doctor or dietitian. You should get advice from a health professional if you are, or are planning to be, pregnant. A dietary supplement of folic acid, for instance, is known to be beneficial.

You don't need to take special vitamin supplements if you eat a healthy and varied diet.

If you do take vitamins or supplements of any kind, make sure you do not exceed the recommended dose – there can be risks in taking large amounts.

Certain drug treatments (e.g. Isoniazid) can deplete the body of vitamins. If you are prescribed these drugs, your doctor will also recommend you take high doses of certain vitamins to compensate. It makes sense to ensure a good intake of essential fatty acids if you have MS.

MANAGING MEALS AND FATIGUE

Preparing meals and snacks can be difficult if you are fatigued, but there are several ways to make things easier for yourself.

Tips for managing fatigue

* Fatigue is a common symptom of MS, so it is important to use your energy wisely, as it can soon run out.
* Take frequent rests.
* Plan ahead.

* Cut out unnecessary tasks.
* Organise space and materials to save energy.
* Learn good postural habits.

In my case, a very hot meal tends to raise my body temperature, causing me to become lethargic. If you are too tired to eat a complete meal, for example, you could eat in two stages (i.e. save your lunch dessert for tea) or eat smaller but more frequent meals. Rather than missing meals, it is worth using convenience foods from time to time, or eating frequent snacks.

Healthy snacks and convenience foods

Fresh fruit is the best convenience food there is – apples, pears, oranges, etc, are full of goodness and easy to eat. Choose starchy foods (carbohydrates) such as cereals, pasta or a baked potato to give you energy, rather than fatty or sweet things. If you eat snacks, beware of processed foods, biscuits and cakes, which can be high in saturated fat and low in nutritional value. If you use ready prepared meals, try things like cottage pie, pasta, curries, or fish cooked in sauce, which are easily available, easy to chew and can be heated in a microwave. Use low fat and low sugar alternatives whenever possible.

* Foods high in carbohydrates will give you energy.
* Snack on fresh fruit.
* Beware of high fat processed foods.
* Look for low fat and low sugar alternatives.
* Better planning will save you time and energy.
* Don't stand when you could sit.
* Organise your kitchen so that utensils and ingredients are within easy reach.
* Labour-saving gadgets can leave you with more time and energy for things you enjoy.

TIPS FOR MANAGING YOUR HEALTH

If you have MS there are a number of ways in which your diet can influence your sense of well being.

Drink plenty of water

Many people with MS experience bladder problems at some point. Ensuring a healthy fluid intake can help minimize the risk of problems or infections.

Some people make the mistake of drinking less liquid to cut down on visits to the toilet, but this can actually make problems worse. Low amounts of concentrated urine encourage infection and irritate the bladder. Low fluid intake can also cause constipation.

There is a limited evidence that a daily intake of one or two glasses of cranberry juice can help reduce urinary tract infections, it won't do you any harm and it tastes good. Large quantities may cause kidney stones, however, so you should never drink more than one litre a day.

The importance of fibre in you diet

Fibre is necessary for a healthy bowel and helps prevent constipation. You should eat a wide variety of high fibre foods daily. The recommended five daily pieces of fruit and vegetables should prevent constipation. Fibre absorbs fluid, so if you increase your fibre intake you should drink more liquids. Talk to your doctor or a continence advisor if you have any problems with your bladder or bowels.

If you are over or underweight

People with MS may lose weight through loss of appetite, or put on weight if they become inactive, and may need to pay particular attention to diet. If you have serious weight problems, your doctor may be able to refer you to a dietitian.

Looking after your skin

The skin is the body's external protective barrier. It is especially important to keep it in good condition if you have mobility difficulties or loss of sensation. A balanced diet and plenty of liquids will help maintain healthy skin, which needs to be well-nourished and supple. Dry, flaky skin is more likely to crack and break down. It can help to use a moisturizing cream or lotion after bathing.

How much you drink, not when you drink, is the important thing.

* Drink 1-2 litres of water or low sugar fluids within every 24-hour period.

* Plan your fluid intake to suit your daily activities.

* Tea, coffee, and alcohol can all increase the need to pass urine, so avoid them if they cause problems.

* Good sources of high fibre foods are: wholemeal bread, wholegrain cereal (e.g. branflakes, porridge, weetabix, and unsweetened muesli), wholewheat pasta, brown rice, beans and pulses, vegetables, fresh and dried fruit.

A diet which is low in saturated fat and high in polyunsaturated fat is the most important part of the self-help management of MS. The diet beneficial for people with MS, advises an increase in all sources of essential fatty acids (EFA), reduce saturated fat and increase 'nutrient dense' food for general good health. There is a wide selection of books about a suitable diet for MS, but as mentioned before, every person is different. You will have to read and decide for yourself, before you start a specialized diet. The following is a quick outline of the foods that should be chosen or avoided on the diet.

CHOOSE

* Fats and Oils-Polyunsaturated margarines, for example sunflower or soya spread and sunflower, corn, safflower. Linseed oil and soya oils should be eaten in moderation. Monosaturates, such as olive oil can be eaten occasionally. Grape seed oil is best to heat.

* Fish-Oily fish such as mackerel, herring, kippers, sardines, whitebait, trout and salmon, should be eaten at least three times a week.

* Meat and Meat Alternatives. Lean Red meat, poultry, game and offal. Try to include 1/4lb of liver, quorn, soya and tofu per week. Aim for only one meat product portion per day (remember this includes cheese.)

* Fruit and Vegetables-Aim for 5 portions a day (1lb.). Fresh fruit and vegetables (fresh or frozen)-particularly salad/raw vegetables and green leafy vegetables. Potatoes-jacket, boiled or mashed and occasionally roasted or homemade chips cooked in suitable oil. Always eat fresh produce whenever possible, ideally organic.

* Pulses-peas, beans, lentils, baked beans, soup made with pulses.

* Grains-Breads (preferably wholemeal), breakfast cereal, porridge, muesli, pasta, rice. Homemade cakes, biscuits and pastries with the appropriate oil. Breadsticks, crispbreads, teacakes, plain biscuits and homemade flapjacks (without coconut) sweetened with a bit of molasses or treacle.

* Dairy Products-Naturally low fat dairy foods. Skimmed milk preferably, or semi-skimmed. Low fat yoghurt, fromage frais, and cottage cheese. Cheese made with polyunsaturated fat (such as 'Flora') in moderation. 'Healthy Eating' sorbet. Hard cheese (preferably half-fat) no more than 1/4lb a week. Eggs (up to 3 or 4 a week.)

AVOID, AVOID, AVOID.

*   Fats and Oils-Frequent fried foods (throw the frying pan away), blended cooking oils, butter, lard, hydrogenated vegetable oils, suet, dripping, low fat spreads, mayonnaise or salad dressings made with saturated fats.

*   Fish - Fried fish (shallow fried in suitable oil may be eaten occasionally), fish in batter, cream sauce, butter or tinned fish in unspecified oil.

*   Meat - Fatty meat, processed meat such as sausages, burgers, corned beef, meat pies, pasties and poultry skin (remove skin and meat fat BEFORE cooking.)

*   Fruits and vegetables - chips, fried vegetables (a stir fry with suitable oil is OK.)

*   Dairy Products - 'Gold Top' milk, full cream, Greek yoghurt, thick and creamy yoghurt and ordinary ice cream.

*   Grains - Muesli with coconut, added vegetable fat, croissants, bought cakes and slimming bars or biscuits.

*   Nuts - Brazils, coconut, cashews, peanuts and peanut butter.

*   Drinks - Try to avoid excessive caffeine.

RAW FOOD DIET

Eating a diet high in natural unprocessed food, which is largely raw and vegetarian, can help in the treatment of the effects of MS. Such a diet can strengthen a weak immune system, which MS sufferers invariably have, and allow the body to attempt to heal itself.

The higher the percentage of raw foods in your diet, the greater your chances of limiting the effects of the illness, as food in its natural organic state is the most compatible with the human body. Switching to a raw food diet may sound daunting but it does not mean going without foods you love. There are raw alternatives to everything from pizza to pasta and what might seem like naughty desserts. You certainly aren't limited to fruits and vegetables. There are many different types of raw food, including herbs, nuts, seeds, grains, spices, beans and pulses.

To prepare the food, you can make a good start with just a blender. A dehydrator helps mimic some cooked food so you can make cookies, bread and crackers without losing the enzymes.

By substantially reducing the amount of toxins entering the body, MS sufferers can expect improvements in their condition. For maximum success, however they need to think about changing their lifestyle and attitude. The body needs as much assistance as it can get to cleanse, renew and strengthen itself. It's also important to seek guidance from an experienced naturopath when making these dietary changes.

The blood type diet

Have diets you've tried in the past failed or even been counter-productive? Are you sure your diet is right for your blood type? This breakthrough new programme, currently sweeping America, is claimed to be the only one to reveal the hidden key to successful dieting. But as explained earlier everybody with MS reacts differently to a particular diet and further scientific proof is required before pinning all your hopes on this new programme.

It claims that your blood type reflects your internal chemistry. It actually determines the way you absorb nutrients. What foods you absorb well and how your body handles stress differ with each blood type. The Eat Right Diet tells you to combine the foods that are right for you:

If your blood type is O:

*   Eat meat (high protein, low carbohydrate)
*   Cut out wheat and most other grains
*   Engage in vigorous aerobic exercise
*   The risk of ulcers and inflammatory diseases such as arthritis increase if you eat incorrectly for your type

If your blood type is A:

*   You should be a vegetarian (high carbohydrate, low fat)
*   Engage in gentle exercise such as yoga or golf
*   Meditate to deal with stress

The risk of cancer and heart disease increase if you eat incorrectly for your type.

If your blood type is B:

*   You should have a very varied diet of all the blood types, one including meat; yours is the only blood type that does well with dairy products.
*   Engage in exercise such as moderate swimming or walking

The risk of slow-growing viruses that attack the nervous system increases if you eat incorrectly for your type

If your blood type AB:

You have most of the benefits and intolerance of types A and B. Engage in calming exercises and relaxation techniques. You have the friendliest immune system of all the blood types

SUPPLEMENTS

The main reason for taking a supplement is because you may be deficient in certain nutrients and by taking supplements you will correct the deficiency. Another good reason for taking supplements is some MS patients have difficulty converting or absorbing certain nutrients.

Evening Primrose Oil - Fatty acids belonging to the linoleic acid family are vital to people with MS, evening primrose is high in gammalinolenic acid – a converted form of linoleic acid. In MS, red blood cells are not only very low in essential fatty acids they are also much bigger than they ought to be, are abnormally shaped, and have a poor ability to regulate the passage of fluids through cell membranes. Evening Primrose Oil can correct this defect within a matter of months. Recommended dosage for MS patients is a 500mg capsules six times a day.

Cod Liver Oil - Fish oils contain alpha-linolenic acid, family of essential fatty acids. These oils are used in your brain and your central nervous system. Recommended intake can be found in a diet rich in oily fish or through a cod liver oil supplement.

Vitamin Supplement -T here are good reasons to take supplements of vitamins and minerals. Firstly, your diet may not be supplying enough. Secondly, you may need more than a normal person as you have a chronic illness. Thirdly, some specific vitamins and minerals are vital for the biochemical conversion process of fatty acids. And finally certain vitamins and minerals are essentials if you are taking EFA's to prevent them from oxidation. It is advisable that you discuss supplementation with the Nutritionalist before taking supplements.

> *Healthy this and healthy that, its*
> *good for me and that's a worry.*
> *I would rather have a plate tasty chips*
> *or a bubbling Ruby Murray.*

10 Advice

What am I to do now?
I really do not know how
I don't know where to turn, as money is tight
Oh dear, having MS is one long fight

BENEFITS ADVICE - Nobody ever plans to have MS, and after being diagnosed most people worry about the future and what it will hold for them. Financial worries are a prime area of concern and can be alleviated by finding out what benefits you are entitled to as a disabled person. Many people feel they may be tempting fate by accessing benefits, but I believe it is never too early to find out what you are entitled to.

Insurance

You may discover that the life insurance policy you took out ages ago insures you against a chronic condition like MS. It is worth your time to pull out the policy and read it over. There are benefit advisors that can help you decipher insurance jargon, make inquiries on your behalf, and fill out any forms necessary for a claim.

Incapacity Benefit

This is a government benefit paid out to those that are too disabled to work and have paid enough N.I. contributions. This benefit is non-means tested, meaning that you can't be judged upon your savings or partners income, but an occupational pension you receive may reduce your entitlement amount.

People with Multiple Sclerosis commonly access Disability Living Allowance, also known as DLA, as the assessment for eligibility is based upon your level of mobility. DLA, is made up of the care component at three levels and mobility component at two levels.

Higher rate mobility entitles you to access the Motability car scheme. This benefit is also non-means tested, non-taxable and will be paid on top of any other benefits you are claiming. You can receive DLA while in full time employment.

Other benefits

You may be able to access are Income Support, Attendant Allowance, Housing benefit, Council Tax Benefit and Disabled Person's Tax Credit all depending upon your particular circumstances.

Help is there if you only know how
Call the benefits enquiry line right now
Life will be easier with money coming in
To claim a benefit is not a sin

The first step in accessing any benefit is to call the Benefits Enquiry Line 0800 88 22 00 and have the respective benefit application sent out to you (the enquiry line can also advise on your local benefit agency that deal with some benefits.) There is a time limit on returning applications and there are numerous community groups such as DIAL and the CAB that can help with these forms. In the case of some benefits a doctor will be sent to visit you at home to assess your claim. As MS has its good days and bad days (and as Murphy's Law has it the doctor will most likely visit on a good day) it is recommended that you keep a diary of how the disease has affected you. Go over the diary with the doctor and be sure to outline the help that you need, not necessarily the help that you are getting.

If for whatever reason your application is rejected there is an appeal procedure (which has a time limit to file by) please ask for assistance if you find yourself in this situation as there are people to help with the forms and even accompany you to a hearing.

Blue Badges

This parking badge can be accessed through your local social services that will send you a form that will have to be verified by your doctor. The parking badge can be used internationally, so it is helpful to have when renting a car abroad.

Telephone Directory

As a person diagnosed with Multiple Sclerosis you are eligible for free directory assistance. To join this scheme ring 195 and ask for registration, an application will then be sent out to you. The application is brief but must be signed by a GP, nurse or social service employee. Once your application has been received a PIN number will be sent out to you, this must be used every time you use the service. The operator will find numbers you need without hunting through the phone book, and they will also be able to connect you automatically to the requested number.

Disabled Persons Railcard

There is a discount scheme available for disabled passengers, contact your local station or National Railcard Office, The Podium, 1 Eversholt Street, London NW1 1DN

Freedom Pass

Available to disabled people, you must access this through your local social services.

Local Mainstream Health Providers

As much as we would like to be able to we cannot provide all the care necessary for the treatment of Multiple Sclerosis but we can recommend ways accessing local services.

Community Occupational Rehabilitation Services

An occupational therapist (OT) will visit you at your home and can help with a variety of difficulties such as improving mobility, adapting your home to fit your needs, tips and tricks to adjusting to any limitations that MS has created. The OT will work with you to meet your needs and create a tailor made rehabilitation programme. If you require any home adaptations it is your OT that will advise the council of your needs. You must ask your GP for a referral to access community occupational rehabilitation services.

Continence Advisor

A specialized continence advisor is available through your GP or Consultant to provide information about the various ways to deal with any continence problems. It is recommended to see a specialist continence advisor as they have the most up to date methods, drugs and aids to promote continence.

Speech Therapist

Speech, language and swallowing difficulties can be corrected with the help of a speech therapist. You can refer yourself to this service; most speech therapist can be reached through your local hospital.

MS Nurse

Some Consultants have specialized MS Nurses working with them. An MS Nurse can arrange to make a home visit and help you and your family with any questions that you may have about MS. This service will be arranged through your consultant, if you cannot self refer.

> *I've got my benefits and have my money,*
> *I drive a car but at times its not that funny,*
> *When I find some arsehole has a blue badge space,*
> *If I had the strength they would get a punch in the face.*

11 Religious Faith

This is the testimony of Silvia Quirk.

My life seemed pretty ordinary, just line everyone else's. I was brought up in a Christian family and was sent to Sunday school as a young girl, but this fell away when I reached 13. This was because I was very shy and afraid to join in as most of my friends had left too. I stilled believed in god, praying at night and mainly when I was frightened. I had many fears in my young life.

Things started to change after my marriage and the birth of my two children, when I was suddenly struck down with severe back pain. I was a very active person loving and living life to the full, always out doing something, disco's, walking, so it came as a bit of a shock to me when I found it extremely difficult to do the things took for granted. Shopping became a hard slog, standing making meals was extremely painful and at night, I had to crawl on my hands and knees to bed.

Mornings were the worsted, as I couldn't get out of bed due to stiffness and pain. This led me to feel down and depressed because of the constant pain and discomfort.

My doctor prescribed painkillers which didn't really help much, then came the bombshell, its osteoarthritis, I was only young and didn't know what the future held for me. I was feeling very sorry for myself, but most of all angry that something like this had happened to me, WHY ME?

I sent my children to Sunday school just as I had been, I only went my self on special occasions as I really didn't think much about God at the time. One day they asked me to support them at church, as they will be carrying the guide flag and it would make them proud if I was there. It was at this service that there were prayers for healing and I thought about going up to be blessed. I was a bit afraid and thought what can

God do for me, can he help in any way? But my children were saying go on Mam, he might be able to heal your back and you will be better. So I plucked up the courage and stepped forward, I thought I would try anything to get rid of this pain.

There was a curate there who laid his hands on my head and prayed for me and then he anointed me with oil. I somehow felt different, there was a numbness in my back and I felt exited, like a full of joy feeling that I had never felt before. I had very little faith and only tried it as a last resort, nothing ventured nothing gained so to speak.

With this new feeling in my body, I seemed to know that God had reached out to my broken body and brought me to him. I was amazed, but still had this feeling that the pain would come back, but thanks be to God it never has. I still suffer arthritis in my body, but now I have someone who is with me always and helps me through the difficult days and uplifts my spirit. Then I started to want to know more about a god who con bring peace in the midst of suffering. He is everything to me now, I love him and worship him and I will never turn my back on him again.

I started to read the bible every day and now spend time with him in pray and meditation. My life feels fulfilled now as he has taken a lot of fear away from my life, which seemed to bind me up in chains. I started to be more confident the more I put trust in him, my fear of the dark disappeared, as I asked Jesus to comfort me in bed. I have conquered my fear of flying and now travel all over the world, thanks to his presence as he gives me more and more everlasting love. My confidence has grown, my shyness has gone and what a joy it is to talk to everyone, even strangers.

Today I met Colin at the swimming baths and as we chatted about faith I realised that all my fears were a thing of the past. He asked if I would put something about faith in writing, so he might understand more and include it in the book he was writing about a life with MS. I pray for all people with MS that this testimony will encourage them to seek out the lord who can help in all circumstances. I feel that it was a privilege that the lord brought Colin along my path and that I was able to discuss my faith with him. God bless you all.

Passages in the bible have helped me in the past years and now help me look to the future what ever that might hold. Zachariah chapter 10 verse 12, strong in the lord. Matthew chapter 10 verse 31, he knows everything about us because he made us, so don't be afraid. Isaiah chapter 49 verse 16, he has written your name on the palm of his hand.

Psalm 121, for protection and fear.

Jesus is my friend, he never lets me down, he's always their for me, even when I do wrong he forgives me. Jesus died for me so I can have eternal life with him, to be with God forever. In this life he has left me a helper, the holy spirit, who comforts me when I am ill and sad. I invite the wholly spirit into my heart and the peace comes, he also gives me confidence to do his work. I am telling others about him, taking care of the sick by supporting them with pray and encouragement. Give your life, your day to Jesus if you haven't already done so, he listens to us every minuet of every day.

God bless you all.
Silvia Quirk

The Endings

So here we are, after your travel through my thoughts, deeds trials and tribulations. I hope it has been pleasant, informative and sometimes humorous, because if you can't laugh at yourself as you go through the same mistakes as me, then you will probably worry yourself to death. Don't let MS grind you down, or you will stay down.

Colin Biggs

USEFUL PHONE NUMBERS AND ADDRESSES

Federation of Multiple Sclerosis Therapy Centre,
Bradbury House, 155 Barkers Lane, Bedford, MK4 9RX
Tel: 0123 432 5781

The MS Research Trust,
Spirella Building, Bridge Road, Letchworth, Hertfordshire, SG6 4ET
Tel: 01462 476700
www.msresearchtrust.org.uk"   www.msresearchtrust.org.uk

The Multiple Sclerosis Resource Centre,
7 Peartree Business Centre, Peartree Road, Stanway, Colchester, CO3 5JN
Tel: 01206 505444
"mailto:themsrc@yahoo.com"   themsrc@yahoo.com

Multiple Sclerosis Society,
372 Edgeware Road, London, NW2 6ND
Tel: 020 8438 0700   Helpline: 0808 800 8000   www.mssociety.org.uk

Benefits Enquiry Line   Tel: 0800 88 22 00

RADAR (The Royal Association for Disability and Rehabilitation),
12 City Forum, 250 City Road, London, EC1V 8AF
Tel: 0207 250 0212   www.radar.org.uk"   www.radar.org.uk

DIAL (Disabled Information and Advice Line
1a Warner Road, Walthamstow, London, E17 7DY   Tel: 0208 520 4111

The National Institute of Conductive Education
Cannon Hill House, Russel Road Birmingham, B13 8RD
www.conductive-education.org   www.conductive-education.org

BIBLIOGRAPHY/REFRENCES

The Lancet 2002 359:1221-31
Prof Alastair Compston FRCP-Prof Alistair Coles MRCP
www.mult-sclerosis.org/news/may2002

National Academy Press
Multiple Sclerosis (2001) Characteristics and Management of Symptoms
www.books.nap.edu

Conductive Education (web site)
www.conductive-education.org

MS Therapy Centres's (web site)
ms-selfhelp.org

Hyperbaric Oxygen Therapy
www.mstherapycentres.org.uk/about-hbo.htm"

Global Health Trax
Hydroxygen Plus
mysiteinc.com/mnmlmru/trax.html
www.biomedx.com/hydroxygen"

Science Daily Magazine
Second patient with MS, undergoes groundbreaking surgery at Yale
www.sciencedaily.com/releases"

Clair Garner
Daily Express-Woman August 26, 2002

The Eat Right Diet
Dr Peter D'Adamo with Catherine Whitney

MS Healing Trust
Dolphin newsletter March 2002   www.msht.org" www.msht.org

Sunday Telegraph
January 29th 2006, page 25

MS Society Publications
MS on your MIND
Dr Caroline Young, Dr Kieran O'Driscoll, Dr Everard Thornton
Spring 2001

Treating MS Symptoms
Gill Roberts
Winter 2000

MS and Healthy Eating
Mala Bhinda, Elaine Hill, Bernadette Porter,
Antthea Masarei and Jo Balcombe.
National Hospital for Neurology & Neurosurgery
Summer 1998

Growing Younger with Yoga
Louise Wiggins
Grange Books 2001

The Multiple Sclerosis Resource Center
Bi Monthly Magazine PATHWAYS
(More so called remedies than there is stars in the sky) but a good read never
the less and one I suggest you order.

THE YOUNG ONES

Stories for emerging adults about the wonderful new world they are about to enter is not what they expect ...

'No Cuddles Today' by Jackie Kain   *ISBN 978-1-902628-62-2*
The moving story of a girl, physically abused in childhood, and how she came to terms with life.

'Broken Wings' by Katherine Munro   *ISBN 978-1-902628-65-3*
The moving story of a girl, mentally abused in childhood, and how she lost her health but maintained her sanity.

'The Russian Girl's Story' by Jeanne Feasey   *ISBN 978-1-902628-63-9*
Separated from her parents during the war in Eastern Europe, the toddler is brought up by the peasant couple who found her.   Later, at the age of eleven, she finds her father is a high-ranking Russian official, in this moving, eye-opening account of human warmth and tragedy.

'A Somerset Childhood' by Phyllis Wyatt   *ISBN 978-1-902628-35-6*
This little girl was poor, but she had a happy childhood in a loving family in a beautiful part of the country. For readers who miss a happy childhood, this childhood is one they can, from within the pages of this book, adopt to fill the gap in themselves.
Hardback edition

'Stay? No Way!' by Vivienne Loranger   *ISBN 978-1-902628-82-0*
When two Australian teenagers run away from their homes, they discover much about the cruel world outside - and much more about their own fickle characters.

Public Library Edition
A comprehensive volume of all the stories published in the Young Ones series is now available for bookshops and public libraries

LOOKING-GLASS COLLECTION

There, with the Grace of God , would go I - a collection of real life stories of ordinary folk in different surroundings, which reveal the extraordinary resilience and range of characteristics of the human personality.

'Present, Miss!' by Frances Lea-Riley   *ISBN 978-1-904494-71-3*
An inspiring and moving story of a successful teacher, for all those who are thinking about joining this worthwhile profession.

'A Teacher's Depression' by Ian Mallon   *ISBN 978-1-904494-11-9*
The personal experiences of a dedicated and caring school teacher coping with work-related stress.

'Nurse, Nurse!' by Nurse Lucy Samuels   *ISBN 978-1-904494-58-4*
The amusing experiences of a dedicated and caring NHS nurse and her patients in hospital.

'Tales out of Church' by the Rev. Andrew Sangster   *ISBN 978-1-904494-11-9*
Few of us knew what lurked behind a cassock until this revealing humorous collection of tales opened our eyes.

'After Virgo ...' by Keith Johnston   *ISBN 978-1-904494-04-1*
Through this work we can share the pain of one diagnosed as having the dreaded disease... and the hopes and fears in the subsequent treatments.

'What's In A Gamble!' by Jake Brindell   *ISBN 978-1-904494-44-7*
The story of a compulsive gambler, and how he gave it up in 100 agonising days. A lesson for us all.

'The Frequent Trader' by Bob Tyson   *ISBN 978-1-902628-34-9*
The story of UK's most successful investor who, without influence, favour, any inside knowledge or previous experience in share dealing, increased the value of his initial savings 68 times its original value in 13 years!

'No Way Out' by Sheila Brookes   *ISBN 978-1-904494-25-6*
For two hours, step inside the shoes of a battered wife and experience her twenty years ordeal.

'Reaching the Light ...' by Linda Rowe   *ISBN 978-1-902628-61-5*
A loving wife's story of how she coped with life andupported her husband as he fought the life-threatening illness of leukaemia - and won.